D1498972

Epidemiology of Drug Abuse

Epidemiology of Drug Abuse

Edited by

Zili Sloboda
Institute for Health and Social Policy
The University of Akron
Akron, OH, USA

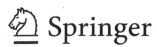 Springer

Library of Congress Cataloging-in-Publication Data

Epidemiology of drug abuse / edited by Zili Sloboda.
    p. cm.
  Includes bibliographical references and index.
  ISBN 0-387-24415-8
  1. Drug abuse–Epidemiology. 2. Drug abuse–Research–Methodology. I. Sloboda, Zili.

  RC564.E65 2005
  362.29–dc22

                                  2005042754

ISBN-10:0-387-24415-8 (Hardbound)   ISBN 0-387-24416-6 (eBook)   Printed on acid-free paper.
ISBN-13:9780387244150

Printed in the United States of America.   (TB/SBA)

9 8 7 6 5 4 3 2 1

springeronline.com

Contributors

Edward M. Adlaf, Centre for Addiction and Mental Health, and Departments of Public Health Sciences and Psychiatry, University of Toronto, Toronto, Ontario, Canada

M. Douglas Anglin, UCLA Integrated Substance Abuse Programs, Los Angeles, California

Mary-Lynn Brecht, UCLA Integrated Substance Abuse Programs, Los Angeles, California

James D. Colliver, Division of Epidemiology, Services and Prevention Research, National Institute on Drug Abuse, Bethesda, Maryland

Kevin P. Conway, Division of Epidemiology, Services, and Prevention Research, National Institute on Drug Abuse, Bethesda, Maryland

Don C. Des Jarlais, Beth Israel Medical Center, New York City, New York

Kirk W. Elifson, Georgia State University, Department of Sociology, Atlanta, Georgia

Samuel R. Friedman, National Development and Research Institutes (NDRI), New York City, New York

Craig Fry, Turning Point Alcohol and Drug Center, Melbourne, Australia and Department of Public Health, University of Melbourne, Melbourne, Australia

Meyer D. Glantz, Division of Epidemiology, Services, and Prevention Research, National Institute on Drug Abuse, Bethesda, Maryland

Paul Griffiths, European Monitoring Centre for Drugs and Drug Addiction, Lisbon, Portugal

Holly Hagan, National Development and Research Institutes (NDRI), New York City, New York

Wayne Hall, Director, Office of Public Policy and ethics, Institute for Molecular Bioscience, University of Queensland, Queensland, Australia

Matthew Hickman, Centre for Research on Drugs and Health Behaviour (CRDHB), Division of Primary Care and Population Health Sciences, Imperial College, London, Great Britain

Yih-Ing Hser, UCLA Integrated Substance Abuse Programs, Los Angeles, California

Robert L. Hubbard, Center for Community-Based Studies, National Development and Research Institutes, Raleigh, North Carolina

Nicholas J. Kozel, Consultant, Bangkok, Thailand

Thomas Locke, University of California, Los Angeles, California

Douglas Longshore, UCLA Integrated Substance Abuse Programs, Los Angeles, California

Rebecca McKetin, National Drug and Alcohol Research Centre, University of New South Wales Sydney, New South Wales, Australia

Michael D. Newcomb, Rossier School of Education, University of Southern California, Los Angeles, California

Jody A. Resko, Dept. of Epidemiology and Population Health, Albert Einstein College of Medicine, Bronx, New York

Claire E. Sterk, Emory University, Rollins School of Public Health, Department of Behavioral Sciences and Health Education, Atlanta, Georgia

Zili Sloboda, Institute for Health and Social Policy, The University of Akron, Akron, Ohio

Colin Taylor, European Monitoring Centre on Drugs and Drug Addiction, Lisbon, Portugal

Carmella Walker, Dept. of Epidemiology and Population Health, Albert Einstein College of Medicine, Bronx, New York

Thomas A. Wills, Dept. of Epidemiology and Population Health, Albert Einstein College of Medicine, Bronx, New York

Preface

The field of drug abuse epidemiology is emergent and its development has been influenced greatly by the stigma attached to the phenomenon of study. Affected populations are often "hidden" and studies of these groups warrant non-traditional epidemiological approaches. For this reason, several unique methods have been developed and tested for sampling, for estimating prevalence, and for studies of general and special populations. A review of available books that include drug abuse epidemiology has revealed a limited perspective that focuses on findings of special studies or on some of the sequelae of drug abuse such as HIV and AIDS. The intent for this book is to provide educators, researchers and the lay public a general overview of the current knowledge within the field of drug abuse epidemiology. It can serve as a supplement to other course offerings in epidemiology, public health, health education or drug abuse. But it also can serve as a general reference for those with an interest in learning more about the field of drug abuse epidemiology.

The structure of the book does not follow the usual format of other epidemiologic texts. The reasoning underlying the structure is the dual intent of the book both as a course text as well as a reference. It covers four major aspects of the field. The first relates to the natural history of drug abusing behaviors and includes a description of the phenomenon, current thinking about origins and pathways as well as etiology of drug use and abuse, the natural history of drug abuse, and the health, social and psychological consequences of drug use and abuse. The second section presents current methodologies used to assess drug abuse within various populations including the use of archival data, sampling methodologies, surveys of general and special populations, indirect methods to estimate prevalence, qualitative techniques applied to drug abuse epidemiology, and the ethics for epidemiologic research. The third section includes descriptive papers summarizing specific studies from the United States and elsewhere that demonstrate the application of these methodologies. The last section gives an overview of the implications of the epidemiology of drug abuse for the prevention and treatment interventions.

Contents

A

Natural History of Drug Abusing Behaviors

1

Defining and Measuring Drug Abusing Behaviors

Zili Sloboda

1. DRUG ABUSE: DEFINING THE PROBLEM

This chapter serves as an introduction to this book and sets the stage for the other chapters that address issues related to the epidemiology of drug abuse. Over the past twenty years drug abuse formerly thought to be a major problem in the United States has become a global challenge. The introduction to a recently published guide to developing a regional integrated information system on drug use captures this idea and the importance of having epidemiological information: "Drug abuse has become a global problem requiring more comprehensive international cooperation to reduce the availability of and demand for drugs. Although

ZILI SLOBODA • Institute for Health and Social Research, The University of Akron drug abuse is becoming an increasing problem for many countries, the experiences to address the problem have been largely those of the more affluent developed countries such as the United States, Canada, Australia, and those in Western Europe. Probably the most important lesson learned by these countries is that to understand their drug abuse problems and to be more efficient in addressing these problems an integrated drug information system is essential. Such a system, if well designed, not only will provide information on the types of drugs being used and the characteristics of those using them but also will generate other more focused studies to provide information that would serve to plan effective prevention and treatment programs." (GAP Toolkit, Module 1, 2003). To develop such an information system that is a useful tool for policy decisions requires addressing key questions regarding the nature of drug abusing behaviors within the socio-political context in which they occur. This chapter lays the groundwork for understanding the relationship between these contextual influences and drug abusing behaviors.

1.1.   What is Drug Abuse?

The terms "drug abuse" or "drug misuse" generally include the use of substances that are considered illegal such as cocaine, heroin, and marijuana, the misuse of legal substances such as solvents, over-the-counter drugs, or prescription drugs, the abuse of tobacco and alcohol, or in the case of underage children, the use of tobacco and alcohol. Most often these substances are used for their psychoactive effects and without the supervision of a physician or other medical professional. The "legal/illegal" labels for these substances are applied through governmental legislation and regulation. In the remainder of this chapter the term "drug" will be used to describe both types of substances.

There has been a longstanding debate over whether drug use is a medical problem or a social problem; over time, it has been recognized as a public health problem. This has become particularly true during the last two decades with the growing recognition of the association of infectious diseases such as HIV/AIDS with drug abuse. There is a dearth of studies on other health consequences of drug use but those that are available show increased negative health effects among drug users. (Andreasson and Allebach, 1995; Cherubin and Sapir, 1993; Fried, 1995; Fried and Watkinson, 2000; Ghodse et al., 1998). It is not often easy to separate those effects that are related to the drugs themselves from the life styles that many drug abusers lead. However unlike other types of health issues, because of the belief in the voluntary nature of drug abuse and misconceptions held about the relative effectiveness of treatment, drug abuse has been highly stigmatized by both policy makers and the general public. As a result, acknowledgement of use or possession of illegal drugs may result in arrest, loss of job, or other sanctions. For these reasons, drug users may be reticent about disclosing drug using behaviors without assurances of confidentiality and trust.

1.2. Definitions

Initially drugs are used voluntarily and primarily for pleasure. It is not clear at what point in the drug-using process biological factors take over and drug abuse or dependence occurs. (Koob et al., 1998; Lyvers, 1998; O'Brien et al., 1998; Tiffany and Carter, 1998; Volkow and Fowler, 2000). The physiological basis of drug abuse and dependence is becoming better understood as our tools for brain imaging improve. Using new brain imaging technologies, such as MRI, PET, and SPECT scans, have enabled researchers to view the living human brain and to note the basic mechanisms involved and mapping what areas are affected by various substances (Volkow et al., 1991; Childress et al., 1995; Altman, 1996) providing explanations for both short- and long-term effects on cognition, memory, and movement (Block and Ghoneim, 1993; Kouri et al., 1999; Pope and Yurgelun-Todd, 1996). However, although these procedures increase our understanding of dependence, the diagnostic tools for measuring and assessing dependence are lacking. Therefore the field has adopted the diagnostic criteria established by psychiatry in the Diagnostic and Statistical Manual of Mental Disorders (DSM). These criteria are specific to individual drugs. The most current edition of DSM (APA, 1994) uses the physiological features of tolerance or withdrawal or, if either is not present, three or more of the following behavioral features: taking larger amounts of the drug over longer periods than intended; experiences of any unsuccessful effort to cut down or control the use of the drug; spending a large amount of time seeking a drug or recovering from its effects; reductions or elimination of important life activities (e.g., job, family); and, continued use of a drug despite persistent or recurrent psychological or physiological problems that are likely to be the result of or exacerbated by the use of the drug. The criteria for drug abuse applies to persons who do not meet the criteria for dependence but have experienced at least one of the following over a 12-month period: recurrent drug use resulting in failure to meet major role obligations (e.g., school, job); recurrent use in physically hazardous situations, recurrent use related legal problems; and, continued use despite persistent or recurrent social or interpersonal problems likely to be the result of or exacerbated by the use of the drug.

Use and abuse/dependence are not just end points of a continuum of drug-using behaviors but represent a number of patterns of use with at the minimum four dimensions: type of drug used, mode of administration, frequency of use, and preferred combinations of drugs used (e.g., cocaine and heroin and marijuana and alcohol). Various researchers may disagree on what other dimensions are involved but all agree that one must initiate the use of drugs before becoming a drug abuser or drug dependent. Therefore, both cross-sectional and longitudinal studies generally ask questions about drug use initiation. These studies show that among those who initiate drug use, only a proportion will progress to abuse or become dependent. This proportion varies, depending on the type of type, frequency of use, and the age at which drug use began (Anthony and Petronis, 1995; Coffey et al., 2000; DeWitt et al., 2000; Fergusson and Horwood, 2000; Grant and Pickering, 1998; Kandel and Chen, 2000; Kandel and Raveis, 1989; Perkonigg et al., 1999).

Dependence measures, adapted from DSM-IV have been included on the National Household Survey on Drug Use and Health (NSDUH; formerly known as the National Household Survey on Drug Abuse). In the 2002 survey, it was estimated that 7.1 million or 1.8 percent of all persons using an illicit drug in the 12 months prior to survey met the survey's dependence classification. These percentages vary by age with the oldest (26 and older) and youngest age groups (12 to 17) having the lowest (1.2 percent through 3.2 percent) while those aged 18 to 25 had the highest percentage considered to be drug dependent, 5.5 percent. (OAS, 2004). Data from longitudinal studies that follow children and adolescents over time have found that adolescents are more likely to become dependent at lower levels of use than adults. (Chen et al., 1997).

While consistent information is available regarding dependence, far less research on the determinants of discontinuation or "natural cessation" of drug use has been reported. The studies that are available have found that adolescents who initiate drug use as a result of social pressures are more likely to stop such use when they mature and take on more adult roles in society.

In summary then, drug using behaviors range from drug use, including any use or misuse of a drug (as defined above), through to drug dependence, associated with either a combination of clinical and behavioral dimensions.

2.   MEASURING DRUG USE AND ABUSE

In the field of epidemiology measurement of a phenomenon generally has two components: the measurement and the means for measurement. For instance, if the epidemiology of hypertension within a community were of interest, then blood pressure would be measured. There are several methods for making these measurements: study subjects could self-report their blood pressure reading from their last medical check up or blood pressures could be measured using a sphygmomanometer. For drug use, there are several biological tests available to test for drug use requiring specimens such as urine, sweat, saliva, and hair. There are both advantages and disadvantages to the use of these tests. The major advantage is that these measures will provide an accurate assessment of the drugs that have been used. A major disadvantage is that it is not always known exactly what drugs are being used and the accuracy of reports depends on the level of sophistication of the study subjects and their familiarity with the drug source. Verebey and Buchan (1997) discuss these techniques in some detail. They summarize by showing the relative advantages and limitations of each biological specimen. The drug detection time varies widely for each from 12–24 hours with saliva and up to 6 months with hair. Furthermore, there are problems with contamination and in collection methods. These tests are appropriate for some populations such as arrestees, pregnant/delivering mothers, or those in treatment where there may be serious repercussions associated with admitting to the use of illicit drugs. In addition, collecting these specimens with large general populations and processing their analysis would be cost-prohibitive; depending on the assay used (e.g., enzyme multiplied immunoassay technique, thin layer chromatography or gas chromatography) and the number of drugs to be detected; these costs can range from one to one hundred dollars. For this reason, the field has depended primarily on self-report. Drug abuse epidemiologists have addressed validity of self-reported drug use extensively. Comparisons of self-reported drug use and the results of biological tests are not consistent and vary by type of drug and by study setting (McNagny and Parker, 1992; Cook and Bernstein, 1994; Fendrich and Xu, 1994; Mieczkowski et al., 1998; Appel, P.W. et al., 2001). For instance, in a drug use survey of 627 residents aged 18 to 40 selected randomly from households in Chicago, Fendrich et al. (2004) found respondents were more likely to report marijuana use than heroin and cocaine. Consolidated drug test results showed that 78 percent of study subjects were found to have used marijuana while only 26 percent and 20 percent of those using heroin and cocaine, respectively, reported use of these drugs on the survey.

Over the three decades in which major population surveys have been conducted within households and schools, researchers have developed procedures that assure a fairly high degree of reliable and valid reporting of substance use (IOM, 1996). There is variation in self-report rates by technique and conditions of the data collection however. (Gfroefer et al., 1997; Lessler and O'Reilly, 1997). For instance, Turner et al. (1997) found that self-administered surveys yield higher rates of illicit drug use than direct or face-to-face interviews. Recent use of computer assisted interviews has demonstrated that this approach not only produces higher reported rates of use but also allows for the rapid transfer of information into a statistical database. In 2000, the Substance Abuse and Mental Health Services Administration's Office of Applied Studies changed the data collection procedures for the NHSDA to a computer-assisted administration. Unfortunately, no methodological studies were conducted to determine differential reporting comparing the face-to-face interview to the new approach.

Accepted measurements for drug using behaviors include at least two measures; type of drug and frequency of use over some time period. Most surveys ask about number of times used over one's lifetime (e.g., have you ever used an illicit drug at least once over your lifetime?), the past 12 months (e.g., have you used an illicit drug at least once in the past year/12 months?), and the last 30 days or past month (e.g., have you used an illicit drug at least once in the past month/30 days?). For some drugs of interest, if respondents report past 30 day use, they will be asked about the number of days in the past 30 days that they used the drug to get an estimate of daily use.

In addition, for respondents reporting any lifetime use of a drug, most surveys will ask respondents about the age when they first used the drug. This information provides estimates of age of initiation and when a survey is conducted on a regular basis over time, differences in the reported age of initiation provides good age-cohort information showing how public attitudes toward drug use may be related to actual use.

3.   IMPLICATIONS FOR EPIDEMIOLOGIC STUDIES

Reasons for making an assessment of drug use within a community or a nation may include the need to understand the types of drugs being used and the extent and pattern of such use and to monitor the emergence of new drugs of abuse or new forms of old drugs (e.g., powder cocaine and crack-cocaine), new administration patterns (e.g., smoking, snorting, inhaling, oral ingestion, injecting), or new population groups at risk for drug use (e.g., younger, higher socio-economic status, ethnicity). The health risks such as the spread of HIV from injecting drug users to the general population may prompt special epidemiologic studies.

In general, epidemiologic studies can address such questions as:

- How pervasive is substance use and abuse in our community/nation?
- Who requires treatment?
- What substances are being used and how are they used?
- What are the characteristics of those involved in such use?
- What factors seem to be associated with substance use and abuse? Do these factors differ for initiation of use from those associated with continued use?
- What circumstances in our community/nation seem to be associated with changing trends in substance use?
- What are the health, social, and psychological consequences of such use for affected individuals, their families and our community/nation?

The diversity of these questions and the means to develop the data bases needed to answer them requires multiple approaches. Generally, these approaches fall under two categories: descriptive epidemiology and analytic epidemiology. The first addresses questions 1–4 while the latter focuses on questions 5–7.

3.1. Descriptive Epidemiology

The measures used in general population surveys of households, students or even groups of drug abusers in treatment programs or in jail require "on the ground" information regarding the types of substances used in an area, particularly illicit substance use that includes an array of drugs. For this reason, it is recommended by most epidemiologic methods guides that communities or countries without an extensive amount of information on drug use patterns begin to explore any existing information that is readily available (NIDA, 1998; UNDCP, 2003; WHO, 2000). Such information generally includes any record data from agencies that provide services to drug users (e.g., drug abuse treatment programs, hospital emergency departments or clinics). It is also recommended that groups be formed from members of the community/nation who either specialize or have a strong interest in drug abuse and drug abusers. The United Nations calls these groups an integrated drug information system that brings together those with data or other experiences with drug abusers representing various segments of the community (e.g., law enforcement, treatment, medical services, welfare, research) to review and summarize the available information and to develop plans for future data collection efforts. Even in countries with well-developed epidemiologic data systems, such groups provide information from the "front lines" detecting emergent drug abuse patterns and therefore serve as excellent surveillance systems. A good example of such a group in the United States is the Community Epidemiology Work Group (CEWG) that has been meeting twice a year since 1974 (Sloboda and Kozel, 1999).

This type of information used in conjunction with focus groups of drug abusers or other qualitative studies lays the foundation for the development of population and school surveys. Specifically, the types of drugs that should be included in these surveys are derived from this information. For example, it was through the CEWG that the beginning of the availability of drugs such as crack-cocaine and Rohypnol were detected and included on both the National Household Survey on Drug Abuse and the national school-based survey, the Monitoring the Future Study.

Existing data or qualitative studies although extremely important to define drug use and abuse within a community/nation generally are not population based and therefore have limited utility for developing estimates of the extent of the problem, i.e., incidence and prevalence rates. In order to makes these estimates, a defined population is required and standardized measures used. Household and school surveys that are administered to representative samples of the target population are better able to provide estimates of rates of new (incidence) as well as on-going users of drugs. Chapters in this book by Adlaf and Sloboda, Kozel and McKetin provide additional information about the use of existing information and surveys.

Drug abuse researchers have also developed indirect approaches to estimate the prevalence of drug use (i.e., existing cases) within a geographic area. These approaches which are based on mathematical models that describe the relationship between observed and unobserved members of a group are particularly useful with rare events such as heroin, cocaine or methamphetamine use that are underestimated on population surveys. Examples of these techniques are capture-recapture methods using closed or open populations, back-calculations, multiplier methods, event-based multipliers, modeling multiple indicators (synthetic estimation) and truncated Poisson. (Simeone et al., 2003, Gossop et al., 1994, Wickens, 1993). Each approach has its own limitations as each is based on some registry or listing of people. Comparisons against survey data for defined geographical areas demonstrate higher estimates of abusing populations. The chapter by Hickman and Taylor provides more detailed discussion of these approaches.

Data systems, that include existing record data, qualitative studies, indirect estimation procedures and surveys, when conducted on an ongoing basis, will provide sufficient information to define the drug use problem in a community/nation and to inform policies to address the emergence of new cases (prevention and availability) and to help affected drug users with both their abuse/dependence and related health and social problems (treatment). However support for these systems requires specialized training, manpower and stable funding.

3.2. Analytic Epidemiology

Descriptive information about drug abuse in a community raises questions and generates hypotheses that require more focused study. This type of research is categorized as analytic epidemiology and most of this research addresses the why and how issues of drug abuse. Both quantitative and qualitative methods are used to answer these questions and the combination of methods is becoming more predominant. Qualitative studies may be used for exploratory work to refine the research questions, measurements, criteria for study populations, and data collection procedures. They may also be used to "flesh out" findings from quantitative studies by providing additional information needed to explain unexpected or inconsistent results.

The most common forms of analytic studies are either cross-sectional, longitudinal in design or some combination of both. Most of our knowledge about risk and protective factors comes from studies that follow children or adolescents over several years (e.g., Brook et al., 1997). Special population studies of more at risk groups such as street children, arrestees, the homeless, injecting drug users in or out of treatment, and pregnant women who are drug abusers provide the information on the consequences of drug use to the users themselves and to those associated with them. In most cases data for these populations are collected through questionnaires that may be self-administered or administered by a trained interviewer.

As drug abuse is a highly stigmatized behavior, researchers conducting studies among drug abusers may not always be able to use the more common sampling approaches ordinarily used in other epidemiologic studies. The inclusion of true representation of a particular population in a study when dealing with persons who are highly mobile, such as the homeless, or who wish to remain hidden has required drug abuse researchers to develop alternative approaches to defining the population universe and then selecting and engaging sample subjects from this universe for study. Probably the most well-known approaches for defining the population universe are snow-ball sampling and social network analysis. In general, these approaches begin with selected index cases asking about other people they know that are like them (i.e., use heroin, or who "do drugs" with them). These other individuals are then asked the same questions that were asked of the index case and on and on until available new contacts are exhausted. The listing of all of these contacts forms the universe of subjects and become the foundation against which a sampling frame is applied.

Once a sample is drawn the next challenge is engaging the individual into the study. Consenting procedures that may include tracking information and what to provide as incentives for participation in the study, particularly for on-going, longitudinal studies, must be carefully planned. There are a number of ethical issues related to any research regarding illegal behaviors but for special populations these issues are very sensitive. As indicated above with regards to self-reported substance use, the data collection situation can influence the degree of trust and confidence a study subject will have (Finch and Strang, 1998). Establishing such a relationship from the initial contact with an individual can make continued follow-up much easier. Interview settings should be neutral and private. Researchers need to obtain tracking information that includes relatives and friends or acquaintances of the more difficult to locate study subjects as well as identifying information such as social security numbers. If the researchers believe that they will need to search other records to locate a subject, depending on local laws and institutional review board regulations, specific consents may be required for agencies such as corrections, social service organizations, or the social security administration.

4. CONCLUSIONS

Drug abuse epidemiologists have made great progress in developing method-ologies to measure an elusive public health problem over the past three decades. As we learn more about the biology of dependence, particularly the process of moving from use to addiction, we in the field may be able to refine our own measurements. In addition, as was pointed out by the IOM (1996), there is a great need for more research to examine co-occurring drug use, physical and psychiatric problems, and to continue to refine our methods of data collection and data analyses.

REFERENCES

Altman, J. (1996). A biological view of drug abuse. *Molecular Medicine Today* 2(6), pp. 237–241.

American Psychological Association. (1994). *Diagnostic and Statistical Manual of Mental Disorders*, 4th Edition, American Psychological Association, Washington, D.C.

Andreasson, S. and Allebeck, P. (1990). Cannabis and mortality among young men: a longitudinal study of Swedish conscripts. *Scandinavian Journal of Social Medicine* 18(1), pp. 9–15.

Anthony, J.C. and Petronis, K.R. (1995). Early-onset drug use and risk of later drug problems, *Drug and Alcohol Dependence* 49(1), pp. 9–15.

Appel, P.W., Hoffman, J.H., Blane, H.T., Frank, B., Oldak, R. and Burke, M. (2001). Comparisons of self-report and hair analysis in detecting cocaine use in a homeless/transient sample. *Journal of Psychoactive Drugs* 33(1), pp. 47–55.

Block, R.I., and Ghoneim, M.M. (1993). Effects of chronic marijuana use on human cognition. *Psychopharmacology* 110, pp. 219–228.

Brook, J.S., Balka, E.B., Gursen, M.D., Brook, D.W., Shapiro, J. and Cohen, P. (1997). Young adult's drug use: a 17-year longitudinal inquiry of antecedents. *Psychological Reports* 80(3 Pt. 2), pp. 1235–1251.

Chen, K., Kandel, D.B. and Davies, M. (1997). Relationship between frequency and quantity of marijuana use and last year proxy dependence among adolescents and adults in the United States. *Drug and Alcohol Dependence* 46(1–2), pp. 53–67.

Cherubin, C.E. and Sapira, J.D. (1993). The medical complications of drug addiction and the medical assessment of the intravenous drug user: 25 years later. *Annals of Internal Medicine* 119(10) pp. 1017–1028.

Childress, A.R., Mozley, D., Fitzgerald, J., Reivich, M., Jaggi, J. and O'Brien, C.P. (1995). Limbic activation during cue-induced cocaine craving, *Society for Neuroscience Abstracts* 21(3), p. 1956.

Coffey, C., Lynskey, M., Wolfe, R. and Patton, G.C. (2000). Initiation and progression of cannabis use in a population-based Australian adolescent longitudinal study. *Addiction* 95(11), pp. 1679–1690.

Cook, R.F. and Bernstein, A. (1994). Assessing drug use prevalence in the workplace: A comparison of self-report methods and urinalysis. *International Journal of the Addictions* 29(8), pp. 1057–1068.

DeWit, D.J., Hance, J., Offord, D.R. and Ogborne, A. (2000). The influence of early and frequent use of marijuana on the risk of desistance and of progression to marijuana-related harm, *Preventive Medicine* 31(5), pp. 455–464.

Fenrich, M., Johnson, T.P., Wislar, J.S., Hubbel, A. and Spiehler, V. (2004). The utility of drug testing in epidemiological research: Results from a general population survey. *Addictions* 99(2), pp.197–208.

Fenrich, M. and Xu, Y. The validity of drug use reports from juvenile arrestees. *International Journal of the Addictions* 29(8), pp. 971–985.

Fergusson, D.M. and Horwood, L.J. (2000). Cannabis use and dependence in a New Zealand birth cohort. *New Zealand Medical Journal* 113(1109), pp. 156–158.

Finch, E. and Strang, J. (1998). Reliability and validity of self-report: on the importance of considering context". *Drug and Alcohol Dependence* 51(3), p. 269.

Fried, P.A. (1995). Prenatal exposure to marihuana and tobacco during infancy, early and middle childhood: effects and an attempt at synthesis. *Archives of Toxicology Supplement* 17, pp. 233–260.

Fried, P.A. and Watkinson, B. (2000). Visuoperceptual functioning differs in 9– to 12-year olds prenatally exposed to cigarettes and marihuana. *Neurotoxicology and Teratology* 22(1), pp. 11–20.

Gfroefer, J., Wright, D. and Kopstein, A. (1997). Prevalence of youth substance use: the impact of methodological differences between two national surveys. *Drug and Alcohol Dependence* 47(1), pp. 19–30.

Ghodse, H., Oyefeso, A. and Kilpatrick, B. (1998). Mortality of drug addicts in the United Kingdom 1967–1993. *International Journal of Epidemiology* 27(3), pp. 473–478.

Glantz, M.D. and Pickens, R.W. (1992). Vulnerability to Drug Abuse: Introduction and Overview. In: Glantz, M.D. and Pickens, R.W. (Eds.). *Vulnerability to Drug Abuse*. American Psychological Association, Washington, D.C., pp. 1–14.

Gore, S.M. (1999). Fatal uncertainty: death-rate from use of ecstasy or heroin. *Lancet* 354(186), pp. 1265–1266.

Gossop, M., Strang, J., Griffiths, P., Powis, B. and Taylor, C. (1994). A ratio estimation method for determining the prevalence of cocaine use. *British Journal of Psychiatry* 164(5), pp. 676–679.

Grant, B.R. and Pickering, R. (1998). The relationship between cannabis use and DSM-IV cannabis abuse and dependence: results from the National Longitudinal Alcohol Epidemiologic Survey. *Journal of Substance Abuse* 10(3), pp. 255–264.

Grant, S., London, E.D., Newlin, D.B., Villemagne, V.L., Liu, X., Contoreggi, C., Phillips, R.L., Kimes, A.E. and Margolin, A. (1996). Activation of memory circuits during cue-elicited cocaine craving. *Proceedings of the National Academy of Sciences* vol. 93, pp. 12040–12045.

Kandel, D.B. and Chen, K. (2000). Types of marijuana users by longitudinal course. *Journal of Studies on Alcohol* 61(3), pp. 367–378.

Kandel, D.B. and Raveis, V.H. (1989). Cessation of illicit drug use in young adulthood. *Archives of General Psychiatry* 46(2), pp.109–116.

Koob, G.F., Rocio, M., Carrera, A., Gold, L.H., Heyser, C.J., Maldonado-Irizarry, C., Markou, A., Parsons, L.H., Roberts, A.J., Schulteis, G., Stinus, L., Walker, J.R., Weissenborn, R. and Weiss, F. (1998). Substance dependence as a compulsive behavior. *Journal of Psychopharmacology* 12(1), pp. 39–48.

Kouri, E.M., Pope, H.G., and Lukas, S.E. (1999). Changes in aggressive behavior during withdrawal from long-term marijuana use. *Psychopharmacology* 143, pp. 302–308.

Lessler, J.T. and O'Reilly, J.M. (1997). Mode of interview and reporting of sensitive issues: design and implementation of audio computer-assisted self-interviewing. In: Harrison, L. and Hughes, A. (Eds.), *The Validity of Self-Reported Drug Use: Improving the Accuracy of Survey Estimates*. National Institute on Drug Abuse Research Monograph 167, pp. 366–382.

Lyvers, M. (1998). Drug addiction as a physical disease: the role of physical dependence and other chronic drug-induced neurophysiological changes in compulsive drug self-administration. *Experimental and clinical psychopharmacology* 6(1), pp. 107–125.

McNagny, S.E. and Parker, R.M. (1992). High prevalence of recent cocaine use and the unreliability of patient self-report in an inner-city walk-in clinic. *Journal of the American Medical Association* 267(8), pp. 1106–1108.

Mieczkowski, T., Newel, R. and Wraight, B. (1998). Using hair analysis, urinalysis and self-reports to estimate drug use in a sample of detained juveniles. *Substance Use and Misuse* 33(7), pp. 1547–1567.

National Institute on Drug Abuse. (1998). *Assessing Drug Abuse Within and Across Communities: Community Epidemiology Surveillance Networks on Drug Abuse*. NTIS PB# 98-177496.

O'Brien, C.P., Childress, A.R., Ehrman, R. and Robbins, S.J. (1998). Conditioning factors in drug abuse: can they explain compulsion? *Journal of Psychopharmacology* 12(1), pp. 15–22.

Office of Applied Studies, Substance Abuse and Mental Health Services Administration. (2004). *2002 National Survey on Drug Use and Health, Chapter 8*. http://oas.samhsa.gov/nhsda/2k2nsduh/Results/2k2Results.html#chap8.

Perkonigg, A., Lieb, R., Hofler, M., Schuster, P., Sonntag, H. and Wittchen, H.U. (1999). Patterns of cannabis use, abuse and dependence over time: incidence, progression and stability in a sample of 1228 adolescents. *Addiction* 94(11), pp. 1663–1678.

Pope, H.G., Jr., and Yurgelun-Todd, D. (1996). The residual cognitive effects of heavy marijuana use in college students. *Journal of the American Medical Association* 275(7), pp. 521–527.

Simeone, R., Holland, L. and Viveros-Aguilero, R. (2003). Estimating the size of an illicit-drug-using population. *Statistics in Medicine* 22, pp. 2969–2993.

Sloboda, Z. and Kozel, N.J. (1999). Frontline surveillance: The Community Epidemiology Work Group on Drug Abuse. In M.D. Glantz and C.R. Hartel, (Eds.), *Drug Abuse Origins and Interventions* (pp. 47–62). American Psychological Association, Washington, D.C.

Taylor, R.C., Harris, N.A., Singleton, E.G., Moolchan, E.T. and Heishman, S.J. (2000). Tobacco craving: intensity-related effects of imagery scripts in drug abusers. *Experimental and Clinical Psychopharmacology* 8(1), pp. 75–87.

Tiffany, S.T. and Carter, B.L. (1998). Is craving the source of compulsive drug use? *Journal of Psychopharmacology* 12(1), pp. 23–30.

Turner, C.F. and Miller, H.G. (1997). Monitoring trends in drug use: strategies for the 21st century. *Substance Use and Misuse* 32(14), pp. 2093–2103.

United Nations. (2003). *Developing an Integrated Drug Information System*. V.02-57020.

Verebey, K.G. and Buchan, B.J. (1997). Diagnostic laboratory: screening for drug abuse. In: Lowenstein, J.H., Ruiz, P., Millman, R.B. and Langrod, J.G. (Eds.), Substance Abuse: A Comprehensive Textbook. Williams & Wilkins, Baltimore, Maryland, pp. 369–377.

Volkow, N.D. and Fowler, J.S. (2000). Addiction, a disease of compulsion and drive: involvement of the orbitofrontal cortex. *Cerebral Cortex* 10(3), pp. 318–325.

Volkow, N.D., Fowler, J.S., Wolf, A.P., Hitzemann, R., Dewey, S., Bendriem, B., Alpert, R., and Hoff, A: (1991). Changes in brain glucose metabolism in cocaine dependence and withdrawal. *American Journal of Psychology* 148, pp. 621–626.

Wickens, T.D. (1993). Quantitative methods for estimating the size of a drug-using population. *Journal of Drug Issues* 23, pp. 185–216.

World Health Organization. (2000). *Guide to Drug Abuse Epidemiology*. WHO/MSD/MSB 00.3.

2

Drug Abuse Heterogeneity and the Search for Subtypes

Meyer D. Glantz, Kevin P. Conway and James D. Colliver

1. SUBSTANCE ABUSE AND HETEROGENEITY

Progress in treating health problems is often made by determining the critical commonalities and differences among the phenomena of interest, using observations to discriminate subtypes, and then determining the underlying mechanisms and etiologies of the subtypes. These causal attributions typically become the distinguishing principles on which the sub-categories are based. When the identified subtypes indicate varying etiological factors, there may be varying subtype-specific indicated interventions. In such cases, differential diagnosis then becomes a primary step in formulating optimal treatment. The benefits of specifying the subtypes

MEYER D. GLANTZ, KEVIN P. CONWAY AND JAMES D. COLLIVER • Division of Epidemiology, Services and Prevention Research, National Institute on Drug Abuse, National Institutes of Health of disorders are clear (Glantz and Colliver, 2002). It is much like the difference between selecting a treatment for someone knowing only that they have some condition involving nasal congestion versus selecting a treatment knowing whether they have a cold, the flu, allergies, or a sinus infection. A differential diagnosis would not only improve treatment effectiveness, but it might also help the patient to prevent future episodes by using the information about his or her susceptibilities.

The differentiation of subtypes of psychiatric disorders or the disaggregation of pathological conditions into distinct clinical entities has been an essential step in improving diagnosis and treatment. For example, the delineation of Attention Deficit Disorder (ADD) and in particular its distinction from both a general lack of intellectual aptitude and from willful opposition or laziness has been a major accomplishment. Further differentiation of ADD from ADD co-occurring with Conduct Disorder is also proving to be valuable. Examinations of heterogeneity and subtypes are a central goal in these and other areas of psychopathology research (e.g. McKay et al., 2004; Grilo, Masheb and Wilson, 2001; Spence, 1997). However, the questions as to the extent to which substance abuse is heterogeneous and what is the nature of that heterogeneity are not only unanswered but are often not even addressed.

This is not to suggest that aspects of substance abuse heterogeneity are not recognized. For example, there is no disagreement that people abuse different substances and this is a key factor in their differential diagnosis under the major diagnostic systems, the *Diagnostic and Statistical Manual of Mental Disorders*, (DSM), (APA, 1994) and the *International Classification of Diseases* (ICD), (WHO, 1993). However, there is no consensus about the relationship of these disorder subtypes to each other. For example, there is no consensus on whether alcohol, tobacco, cocaine and heroin dependence are fundamentally the same disorder except for the substance being abused, its legal status, and its physical effects. The other major diagnostic distinction in DSM and ICD relates to the categories of "abuse" and "dependence" for each of the substances covered. Regardless of the distinctions of substance and level of disorder, these diagnostic subcategories serve few of the explanatory or directive functions of fully delineated clinical entities or subtypes.

The issues grow even more complicated given that some researchers hypothesize that substance use disorders arise from common underlying neurochemical systems and responses (e.g. Hyman and Nestler, 1996; Koob and Le Moal, 1997), and others hypothesize that there are common underlying genetic predispositions (e.g. Tsuang et al., 1998; Kendler et al., 2003). There is general agreement that substance abusers are heterogeneous in terms of the drugs they use and the routes of administration, whether they have serious practical and/or psychiatric problems associated with their drug abuse, and whether they are physically (and possibly psychologically) dependent on the drugs they abuse. There is also agreement that abusers often use different drugs at any given time and over time and that they may follow varying patterns of abuse behavior such as having different ages of onset and different patterns of escalation. These observations have not led to any fundamental subcategorization of substance abuse into heuristically useful and distinct clinical entities and there is a tacit assumption of basic underlying homogeneity. Perhaps as a result, the selection of differential treatment is largely based on pharmacological factors and environmental features (such as the legal status of the abused drug) rather than conceptualizations of the fundamental processes involved in substance abuse behavior.

2. EPIDEMIOLOGY

In the general population of the United States 12 years of age and older, around 46 percent—an estimated 108 million individuals—have tried an illicit drug at least once in their lives according to the 2002 National Survey of Drug Use and Health (NSDUH, formerly known as the National Household Survey on Drug Abuse; SAMHSA 2003). Forty percent have tried marijuana and 30 percent have used illicit drugs other than marijuana. Lifetime use of alcohol and tobacco is much higher, with 83 percent indicating they have used alcohol and 73 percent reporting use of tobacco products. One in seven (14 percent) have used cocaine and a similar proportion have tried hallucinogens. One-fifth report having used a prescription-type psychopharmaceutical drug (analgesic, tranquilizer, stimulant or sedative) when they did not have a prescription for it or just for the feeling or experience they expected it would provide. Research has consistently shown that the large majority of those who use drugs do not escalate to substance abuse or dependence (using DSM-IV criteria) suggesting that while the early substance use behaviors may be the same for both those who will and those who will not eventually develop a substance use disorder, the underlying processes may be heterogeneous (Haertzen, Kocher, and Miyasato, 1983; Pomerleau, Pomerleau, Namenek, and Marks, 1999).

Differing patterns of onset and escalation may also be indicative of divergent patterns or subtypes. Individuals who start using drugs early in life are at increased risk of progressing to more serious drugs and of developing drug use disorders (Kandel and Yamaguchi, 1993; Robins and Przybeck, 1985; Anthony and Petronis, 1995; Grant and Dawson, 1998; Lynskey, 2003).

While it cannot be conclusively determined whether early onset, as distinct from correlated factors, accounts for this association, the number of young initiates of some drugs has been increasing in recent years (Figure 1). The top line in this graph shows an increase in new marijuana users who are under 18 years of age from 1990 to 1999, following a decline in the 1980s. New initiates into cocaine use, while not displaying a trend as dramatic as that for marijuana, were more numerous in 2000 than at the height of the cocaine epidemic of the mid-1980s.

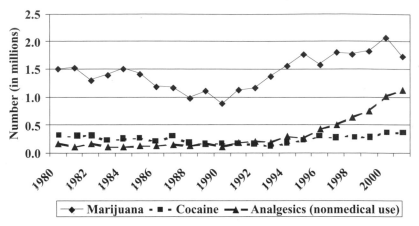

Figure 1. Number of initiates to drug use under age 18 by year and drug.

Of great concern is the recent increase in the number of new nonmedical users of prescription-type analgesics (e.g., oxycodone and hydrocodone).

Drug involvement increases not only through progression from one substance to another (e.g., cigarettes or alcohol to marijuana to other more illicit drugs) but also by escalation in the frequency of use of individual substances, shifts in the patterns and contexts of use, and development of substance abuse and dependence. Table 1 shows data on the frequency of marijuana use and rates of dependence among the estimated 26 million Americans who reported in 2002 that they had used the substance in the past year. Thirty-five percent used marijuana once a month or less, 36 percent used it more than 2 days a week, and 12 percent used it daily or almost daily (SAMHSA, 2003a). The likelihood of dependence on a drug increases with frequency of use. Among all past-year marijuana users, around 10 percent met Diagnostic and Statistical Manual of Mental Disorders, Fourth Edition (DSM-IV; APA, 1994) criteria for dependence on the drug in that time frame. As shown in Table 1, less than 5 percent of those who used marijuana two days a month or less often reported symptoms that met dependence criteria; among those using it daily or almost daily in the past year, however, 26 percent were dependent. Similar findings were reported by Grant and Pickering (1998).

The proportion of substance users who become dependent varies by drug. Estimates from the National Comorbidity Survey (NCS) indicated that 15 percent of lifetime alcohol users are dependent on alcohol at some time in their lives (Anthony et al., 1994). As shown in Figure 2, higher rates of lifetime dependence among lifetime users are found with tobacco (32 percent), heroin (23 percent), and cocaine (17 percent), while lower rates are observed with stimulants (11 percent), anxiolytics (9 percent), cannabis (9 percent), and analgesics (8 percent). These figures are for 1990–1992 and are based on individuals 15–54 years of age.

Table 1. Frequency of Marijuana Use and Its Association with Dependence: 2002

Days used in past year	Percent of past-year users	Percent meeting criteria for dependence in past year
1 to 12 days	34.5	0.3
12 to 24 days	11.9	4.2
25 to 50 days	7.5	10.6
51 to 100 days	10.0	11.3
101 to 200 days	14.5	15.3
201 to 300 days	9.7	23.8
301 to 365 days	11.8	26.2
Overall	100.0	10.2

Source: 2002 National Survey of Drug Use and Health, Substance Abuse and Mental Health Data Archives Online Data Analysis System.

Also part of the question of the relationship of substance use to abuse and dependence are the questions of whether, and under what conditions, substance use is effectively equivalent to sub-threshold abuse or dependence. Similar questions have been raised related to models of other psychopathologies and have led to advances in understanding those disorders (e.g. for a discussion on sub-threshold depression, see Cuijpers and Smit, 2004). Investigating the heterogeneity of substance use patterns might lead to improved identification of those likely to experience significant problems even if their substance use does not escalate as well as early identification of those at greatest risk for experiencing significant problems associated with substance use escalation.

Scientific recognition that use, abuse and dependence are not just points on a continuum has been important. It has led, for example, to research showing that the predisposing or risk factors for drug use are different than those for abuse,

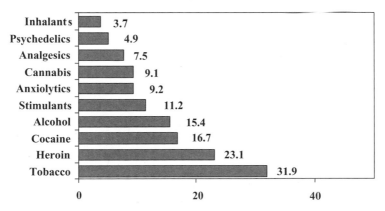

Figure 2. Rate of lifetime dependence among lifetime users 15 to 44 years old, by drug.

(Glantz and Pickens, 1992). Further investigations of the risk factors for substance use disorders might also help to explicate its heterogeneity and to suggest possible subtypes.

3. RISK FACTORS

Research has identified a wide range of risk factors for drug use and drug abuse (e.g. Hawkins et al., 1992) and some protective factors have also been identified. However, there have been few attempts to investigate these risk factors to determine if they group in meaningful clusters and to explore whether they are associated with subtypes of substance use disorders or even if they are specific only to substance use. Risk factors for substance use are often not distinguished from risk factors for substance use disorders, and it is often assumed that risk factors for substance involvement accumulate in a relatively linear fashion. While a greater number and severity of risk factors are likely to be associated with a higher-level risk and severity of outcome, different clusters of risk factors may have subtype related implications.

Evidence indicates that there are many paths to substance abuse. However, it is possible that the use of different drugs, differing patterns of drug onset, use and escalation, and/or different risk factors ultimately all converge to the same general substance abuse condition if the case is sufficiently severe. Such a common substance abuse outcome would be an instance of equifinality and if this were the case, then variations in the contributing factors and developmental course might have fewer implications for prevention and differential intervention. Alternatively, if variations in the paths of substance use lead to significantly different subtypes of substance abuse, then distinguishing major variations in etiological factors and patterns would have a wide range of heuristic and intervention implications. If there is such substance abuse multifinality, then it may be the case that significant variations in etiological factors relate to divergent subtypes of substance abuse. However, even if substance abuse is an instance of multifinality, this would not necessarily mean that substance abuse does not have a single underlying process. Such multifinality, if it exists, might result from the interaction of a single underlying process with a diverse range of external factors (e.g. the particular drugs which the individual uses or the protective social influences of the user's family) as well as a wide range of intrinsic factors (e.g. the individual's developmental level or co-occurring psychopathology). In any case, investigating the heterogeneity of etiological factors to identify differing patterns may lead to the identification of substance abuse subtypes and to the explication of their underlying processes. We examined the available research on risk factors for drug abuse to explore this possibility.

Our analysis of current research identified three emergent clusters of risk factors for substance use disorders: behavior disinhibition, affect dysregulation, and conduct disorder/antisocial personality disorder (CD/ASPD) which will be referred to here as antisociality. Converging lines of research have found antisociality to be the most clearly established risk factor(s) for substance use disorders and as such, it will be the focus of this brief review.

3.1. Antisociality

Research shows that antisociality co-occurs with drug abuse, that antisociality confers substantial risk for the various stages of drug involvement ranging from initial drug use to drug dependence, that personality characteristics akin to antisociality are associated with drug abuse, and that the familial diathesis of drug abuse likely involves antisocial behavior and/or personality characteristics that may underlie the behavior.

Research on drug use disorders provides consistent and overwhelming evidence of substantial comorbidity between substance use disorders and antisocial personality disorder (ASPD), characterized by a pattern of irresponsible, impulsive and remorseless behaviors beginning in childhood or early adolescence and continuing into adulthood (APA, 1994). Findings from three large epidemiologic surveys, the Epidemiologic Catchment Area (ECA) survey, the NCS, and the International Consortium in Psychiatric Epidemiology (ICPE) show substantial comorbidity of ASPD with drug abuse and drug dependence (Kessler et al., 2001; Regier et al., 1990; Warner et al., 1995). Indeed, evidence from the ECA survey (Regier et al., 1990) shows that ASPD was the psychiatric disorder with the largest odds-ratio for both alcohol disorders (O.R. = 21.0) and drug disorders (O.R. = 13.4). Most recently, Grant and colleagues have shown that ASPD has markedly strong associations with alcohol and drug abuse and dependence in the general population (Grant et al., 2004). Moreover, the magnitude of comorbidity between antisocial personality disorder and drug involvement has been found to generally increase from drug use to drug dependence (Kessler et al., 1996; Merikangas et al., 1998; Swendsen and Merikangas, 2000). In the NCS, for example, the lifetime risk of adult antisocial behavior was 2.8 for drug abuse and 13.6 for drug dependence (Kessler et al., 1996).

Several studies have shown that the risk attributed to behavior problems increases with the progression from drug use to drug dependence suggesting an etiological link between antisociality and addiction. Robins and McEvoy (1990) reported that the likelihood of substance abuse increases with each conduct problem—a dose-dependent relation that helps support the argument that conduct is a cause of substance abuse problems. Several studies indicate that child psychopathology predicts heavier drug use in adolescence. Focusing on trajectories of drug use from ages 13-18 years, White et al. (2001) found that higher levels of attention-deficit/hyperactivity disorder and conduct disorder predicted higher levels of marijuana use. Lewinsohn et al. (2000) reported that persistent/frequent smoking during adolescence was explained in part by comorbid behavior disorders. Former or current daily smokers, compared to smokers who never smoked on a daily basis, were nearly 4-times as likely to have conduct or oppositional defiant disorder (O.R. = 3.9).

Conduct disorder, the precursor of ASPD that manifests prior to age 16, has also been consistently reported as a risk factor for drug use. In a comprehensive review of fifteen community studies on adolescent substance use and abuse, Armstrong and Costello (2002) reported that behavior disorders were the psychiatric conditions that were most commonly associated with substance abuse. They estimated that substance users or abusers, compared to controls, were four times more likely to have conduct disorder, oppositional defiant disorder, or attention-deficit hyperactivity disorder. Focusing specifically on conduct disorder, several studies have found that this behavior problem is associated with particularly high risk of substance abuse (Armstrong and Costello, 2002; Chilcoat and Bresleau, 1998). The estimates are often higher among clinic samples. Burke, Loeber, and Lahey (2001) reported that conduct disorder was associated with a 6-fold increased risk of tobacco use in a sample of clinic-referred boys.

Aside from the full-blown diagnosis of conduct disorder, several prospective longitudinal investigations reveal childhood externalizing problems as a principal pathway in the development of substance use and substance use disorders (McCord 1981; Robins and McEvoy, 1990). Evidence from community samples includes a follow-up of the Baltimore site of the Epidemiologic Catchment Area survey that indicates that problem behaviors (e.g., fighting, school suspension, frequent lying) prior to the age of 15 was associated with increased risk of injection drug use at approximately 26 years of age (Neumark and Anthony, 1997). Lewinsohn et al. (1995) reported that externalizing behavior problems predicted substance use disorder over a one-year period during adolescence; Reinherz and colleagues (2000) found that hostile/aggressive behavior at age 9 predicted substance use disorder by age 21; and Storr et al. (2004) found that higher levels of teacher-rated childhood misbehavior at entry into primary school were associated with an increased risk of becoming tobacco-dependent by young adulthood. Such findings have helped construct an empirical basis for randomized field trials designed to test hypothesized mechanisms of association. In fact, there is evidence from a randomized study designed to decrease conduct problems that supports an etiologic link between conduct problems and subsequent substance use. Kellam and Anthony (1998) found that boys who were assigned to a 2-year behavior-improving classroom program, compared to boys assigned to usual classroom environments, were less likely to begin smoking cigarettes in early adolescence. In short, converging lines of evidence indicate that substance abuse and antisocial behavior are intimately connected problems of significant concern to public health.

It is likely that antisociality will be important in interpreting the well-established finding that a positive family history of substance abuse confers substantial risk for substance use outcomes. Although controlled family studies demonstrate that drug disorders run in families (Bierut et al., 1998; Merikangas et al., 1998) and twin and adoption studies (Pickens et al., 1991; Grove et al., 1990; Jang et al., 1995; Tsuang et al., 1998; Kendler et al., 1999; Kendler et al., 2000) show that the familial clustering of drug abuse can be explained in part by genetic factors, the specific processes through which familial drug abuse exerts an influence is not clear. Evidence suggests that greater research attention to psychiatric comorbidity, particularly comorbid antisociality, may inform our understanding of such processes. Cadoret's classic adoption studies have suggested, for example, that the role of genetic factors in the development of drug abuse involves two paths from parent to adopted-away offspring. The first path indicates a direct association between substance abuse in the biologic parent and drug abuse in the adoptee. The second path indicates an association from antisocial personality disorder in the biologic parent to aggressive behavior in the adoptee, which in turn is associated with drug abuse in the adoptee (Cadoret, 1992; Cadoret et al., 1986; Cadoret et al., 1996).

There is some support for the notion that antisociality operates as a moderator for family history of drug abuse. Relying on follow-up data from Cadoret's sample, Langbehn and colleagues (2003) applied survival analyses methodology to age-of-onset data for both drug use and drug disorders in an attempt to examine whether family history of drug abuse with antisocial personality disorder poses greater risk than family history of drug abuse without antisocial personality disorder. When predicting both drug use and drug disorders in adoptees as young adults, results showed that the presence of drug abuse combined with antisocial personality disorder in the adoptee's biological father increases the risk for the development of drug problems in the adoptee. Similar findings have been reported in other samples. Moss and colleagues (2002) showed that adolescent offspring of fathers with substance dependence (with or without antisocial personality disorder) faired worse than those without substance dependence on several measures of family functioning. Yet, children of fathers with both substance dependence and antisocial personality disorder demonstrated the highest levels of externalizing and internalizing psychopathology as well as greater affiliation with deviant peers which, in turn, was associated with psychopathology. Chassin and colleagues (2002) found that adolescent offspring of alcoholics with comorbid antisocial personality disorder, compared to offspring of alcoholics only, were more likely to be classified into the high-risk group characterized by early and heavy drinking patterns.

4.   CONCLUSIONS

In addition to the research on the association between substance use disorders and antisociality, there is a large body of literature reporting connections with behavior disinhibition and affect dysregulation. It is not possible in this short chapter to review these and other findings on risk factors for substance use disorders. However, the above discussion illustrates the convergences in the research findings on risk factors that point to possible clusters having implications for further understanding the heterogeneity of substance abuse and the identification of drug abuse subtypes.

It is also not possible in this chapter to discuss important related issues, such as the relationship of heterogeneity to substance use disorder phenotypes and endophenotypes, the role of protective factors in the divergence of subtypes, the relationship of co-morbid psychiatric conditions and developmental psychopathology to heterogeneity, developmental influences, and individual and group diversity, and the implications of heterogeneity and subtypes for prevention and treatment. Despite the unanswered questions, however, it is clear that investigation of the heterogeneity of substance use disorders and their underlying processes can advance our ability to effectively understand, prevent and treat substance abuse.

It is clearly important to go beyond the recognition of the heterogeneity of drug abuse and to look for systematic variations in the etiology and manifest patterns of substance abuse. There may be critical variations in the underlying processes of substance abuse as well as significant systematic differences in the observable behavior patterns. Distinguishing major divergences in the differing patterns may lead to the identification of clinically significant subtypes, help determine the underlying processes of substance abuse, and facilitate the study of the ways in which environmental factors interact with individuals' characteristics (and the underlying processes of substance abuse) to result in different subtypes. While the available research does not answer the question of whether there are drug abuse subtypes, it does provide encouragement to continue the search.

Disclaimer. The views expressed in this article do not necessarily represent the National Institutes of Health or the Department of Health and Human Services.

REFERENCES

American Psychiatric Association. (1994). *Diagnostic and Statistical Manual of Mental Disorders— Fourth Edition.* American Psychiatric Association, Washington, D.C.

Armstrong, T.D. and Costello, E.J. (2002). Community studies on adolescent substance use, abuse, or dependence and psychiatric comorbidity. *Journal of Consulting and Clinical Psychology* 70, pp. 1224–1239.

Anthony, J.C., Warner, L.A., and Kessler, R.C. (1994). Comparative epidemiology of dependence on tobacco, alcohol, controlled substances, and inhalants: Basic findings from the National Comorbidity Survey, *Experimental and Clinical Psychopharmacology* 2, pp. 224–268.

Anthony, J.C. and Petronis, K.R. (1995). Early-onset drug use and risk of later drug problems. *Drug and Alcohol Dependence* 40, pp. 9–15.

Babor, T.F., Hofmann, M., DelBoca, F.K., Hesselbrock, V., Meyer, R.E., Dolinsky, Z.S. and Rounsaville, B. (1992). Types of alcoholics, I. Evidence for an empirically derived typology based on indicators of vulnerability and severity. *Archives of General Psychiatry* 49, pp. 599–608.

Bierut, L.J., Dinwiddie, S.H., Begleiter, H., Crowe, R.R., Hesselbrock, V., Nurnberger, J.I. Jr., Porjesz, B., Schuckit, M.A., and Reich, T. (1998). Familial transmission of substance dependence: Alcohol, marijuana, cocaine, and habitual smoking: A report from the Collaborative Study on the Genetics of Alcoholism. *Archives of General Psychiatry* 55, pp. 982–988.

Burke J.D., Loeber R. and Lahey, B.B. (2001). Which aspects of ADHD are associated with tobacco use in early adolescence? *Journal of Child Psychology and Psychiatry* 42, pp. 493–502.

Cadoret, R.J. (1992). Genetic and environmental factors in initiation of drug use and the transition to abuse. In M. Glantz and R. Pickens (Eds.), *Vulnerability to Drug Abuse*. American Psychological Association, Washington, D.C., pp. 99–113.

Cadoret, R.J., Yates, W.R., Troughton, E, Woodworth G. and Stewart MA. (1996). An adoption study of drug abuse/dependency in females. *Comprehensive Psychiatry* 37, pp. 88–94.

Cadoret, R.J., Troughton, E., O'Gorman, T., and Heywood, E. (1986). An adoption study of genetic and environmental factors in drug abuse. *Archives of General Psychiatry* 43, pp. 1131–1136.

Chassin L, Pitts S.C., and Prost, J. (2002). Binge drinking trajectories from adolescence to emerging adulthood in a high-risk sample: predictors and substance abuse outcomes. *Journal of Consulting and Clinical Psychology* 70, pp. 67–78.

Chilcoat, H.D. and Breslau, N. (1998). Posttraumatic stress disorder and drug disorders: Testing causal pathways. *Archives of General Psychiatry* 55(10), pp. 913–917.

Cuijpers, P. and Smit, F. (2004). Subthreshold depression as a risk indicator for major depressive disorder: a systematic review of prospective studies. *Acta Psychiatrica Scandinavia* 109, pp. 325–331.

Glantz, M.D. and Colliver, J.D. (2002). Drug use, drug abuse, and heterogeneity. *Bulletin on Narcotics*, United Nations 54(1), pp. 45–59.

Glantz, M.D., and Pickens, R.W. (1992). Vulnerability to drug abuse: Introduction and overview. In M. Glantz and R. Pickens (Eds.), *Vulnerability to drug abuse*. American Psychological Association, Washington, D.C., pp. 1–14.

Grant, B.F. and Dawson, D.A. (1998). Age of onset of drug use and its association with DSM-IV drug abuse and dependence. *Journal of Substance Abuse* 10, pp. 163–173.

Grant, B.F. and Pickering, R. (1998). The relationship between cannabis use and DSM-IV cannabis abuse and dependence: Results from the National Longitudinal Alcohol Epidemiologic Survey. *Journal of Substance Abuse* 10(3), pp. 225–264.

Grant, B.F. Stinson F.S., Dawson, D.A., Chou, S.P., Ruan, W.J., and Pickering, R.P. (2004). Co-occurrence of 12-month alcohol and drug use disorders and personality disorders in the United States: Results from the National Epidemiologic Survey on Alcohol and Related Conditions. *Archives of General Psychiatry* 61, pp. 361–368.

Grilo, C.M., Masheb, R.M., and Wilson, G.T. (2001). Subtyping binge eating disorder. *Journal of Consulting and Clinical Psychology* 69(6), pp. 1066–1072.

Grove, W., Eckert, E., Heston, L., Bouchard, T., Segal, N., and Lykken, D. (1990). Heritability of substance abuse and antisocial behaviour: A study of monozygotic twins reared apart. *Biological Psychiatry* 27, pp. 1293–1304.

Haertzen, C.A., Kocher, T.R., and Miyasato, K. (1983). Reinforcements from the first drug experience can predict later drug habits and/or addiction: results with coffee, cigarettes, alcohol, barbiturates, minor and major tranquilizers, stimulants, marijuana, hallucinogens, heroin, opiates and cocaine. *Drug and Alcohol Dependence* 11, pp. 147–165.

Hawkins, J.D., Catalano, R.F., and Miller, J.Y. (1992). Risk and protective factors for alcohol and other drug problems in adolescence and early adulthood: Implications for substance abuse prevention. *Psychological Bulletin* 112(1), pp. 64–105.

Hyman, S.E. and Nestler, E.J. (1996). Initiation and adaptation: a paradigm for understanding psychotropic drug action. *American Journal of Psychiatry* 153, pp. 151–162.

Jang, K.L., Livesley, W.J., and Vernon, P.A. (1995). Alcohol and drug problems: a multivariate behavioural genetic analysis of co-morbidity. *Addiction* 90, pp. 1213–1221.

Kandel, D.B. and Yamaguchi, K. (1993). From beer to crack: Developmental patterns of drug involvement. *American Journal of Public Health* 83(6), pp. 851–855.

Kellam, S.G. and Anthony, J.C. (1998). Targeting early antecedents to prevent tobacco smoking: Findings from an epidemiologically based randomized field trial. *American Journal of Public Health* 88, pp. 193–197.

Kendler K.S., Jacobson K.C., Prescott C.A., and Neale M.C. (2003). Specificity of genetic and environmental risk factors for use and abuse/dependence of cannabis, cocaine, hallucinogens, sedatives, stimulants, and opiates in male twins. *American Journal of Psychiatry* 160(4), pp. 687–695.

Kendler, K.S., Karkowski, L.M., and Prescott, C.A. (1999). Hallucinogen, opiate, sedative and stimulant use and abuse in a population-based sample of female twins. *Acta Psychiatrica Scandinavia* 99, pp. 368–376.

Kendler, K.S., Karkowski, L.M., Neale, M.C., and Prescott, C.A. (2000). Illicit psychoactive substance use, heavy use, abuse and dependence in a US population-based sample of male twins. *Archives of General Psychiatry* 57, pp. 261–269.

Kessler, R.C., Aguilar-Gaxiola, S., Andrade, L., Bijl, R., Borges, G., Caraveo-Anduaga, J.J., DeWit, D.J., Kolody, B., Merikangas, K.R., Molnar, B.E., Vega, W.A., Walters, E.E., Wittchen, H.U., and Ustun, T.B. (2001). Mental-substance comorbidities in the ICPE surveys. *Psychiatria Fennica* 32 (suppl 2), pp. 62–79.

Kessler, R.C., Nelson, C.B., McGonagle, K.A., Edlund, M.J., Frank, R.G., and Leaf, P.J. (1996). The epidemiology of co-occurring addictive and mental disorders: Implications for prevention and service utilization. *American Journal of Orthopsychiatry* 66, pp. 17–31.

Koob, G.F. and Le Moal, M. (1997). Drug abuse: hedonic homeostatic dysregulation. *Science* 278(5335), pp. 52–58.

Langbehn, D.R. and Cadoret, R.J. (2001). The adult antisocial syndrome with and without antecedent conduct disorder: Comparisons from an adoption study. *Comprehensive Psychiatry* 42, pp. 272–282.

Lewinsohn, P.M., Brown, R.A., Seeley, J.R., and Ramsey, S.E. (2000). Psychosocial correlates of cigarette smoking abstinence, experimentation, persistence and frequency during adolescence. *Nicotine and Tobacco Research* 2, pp. 121–131.

Lewinsohn, P.M., Gotlib I.H., and Seeley, J.R. (1995). Adolescent psychopathology: IV. Specificity of psychosocial risk factors for depression and substance abuse in older adolescents. *Journal of the American Academy of Child and Adolescent Psychiatry* 34, pp. 1221–1229.

Lynskey, M.T., Health, A.C., Bucholz, K.K., Slutskey, W.S., Madden, P.A., Nelson, E.C., Stratham, D.J., and Martin, N.G. (2003). Escalation of drug use in early onset cannabis users vs. co-twin controls. *Journal of the American Medical Association* 289, pp. 427–433.

McKay, D., Abramowitz, J.S., Calamari, J.E., Kyrios, M., Radomsky, A., Sookman, D., Taylor S. and S. Wilhelm. (2004). A critical evaluation of obsessive-compulsive disorder subtypes: Symptoms versus mechanisms, *Clinical Psychology Review* 24(3), pp. 283–313.

Merikangas, K.R., Mehta, R.L., Molnar, B.E., Walters, E.E., Swendsen, J.D., Aguilar-Gaziola, S., Bijl, R.V., Borges, G., Caraveo-Anduaga, J.J., DeWit, D.J., Kolody, B., Vega, W.A., Wittchen, H.U., and Kessler, R.C. (1998). Comorbidity of substance use disorders with mood and anxiety disorders: Results of the international consortium in psychiatric epidemiology. *Addictive Behaviors* 23, pp. 893–907.

Merikangas, K.R., Stolar, M., Stevens, D.E., Goulet, J., Priesig, M., Fenton, B., and Rounsaville, B.J. (1998). Familial transmission of substance use disorders. *Archives of General Psychiatry* 55, pp. 973–979.

Moss, H.B., Lynch, K.G., Hardie, T.L., and Baron, D.A. (2002). Family functioning and peer affiliation in children of fathers with antisocial personality disorder and substance dependence: associations with problem behaviors. *American Journal of Psychiatry* 159, pp. 607–614.

Neumark, Y.D. and Anthony, J.C. (1997). Childhood misbehavior and the risk of injection drug use. *Drug and Alcohol Dependence* 48, pp. 193–197.

Pomerleau, C.S., Pomerleau, O.F., Namenek, R.J., and Marks, J.L. (1999). Initial exposure to nicotine in college-age women smokers and never-smokers: a replication and extension. *Journal of Addictive Disorders* 18, pp. 13–19.

Regier, D.A., Farmer, M.E., Rae, D.S., Locke, B.Z., Keith, S.J., and Judd, L.L. (1990). Comorbidity of mental disorders with alcohol and other drug abuse: Results from the Epidemiologic Catchment Area (ECA) study. *Journal of the American Medical Association* 262, pp. 2511–2518.

Reinherz, H.Z., Giaconia, R.M., Hauf, A.M., Wasserman, M.S., and Paradis, A.D. (2000). General and specific childhood risk factors for depression and drug disorders by early adulthood. *American Academy of Child and Adolescent Psychiatry* 39, pp. 223–231.

Robins, L.N. and McEvoy, L. (1990). Conduct problems as predictors of substance abuse. In L. Robins and M. Rutter (Eds.), *Straight and Deviant Pathways from Childhood to Adulthood*. New York: Cambridge University Press, pp. 182–204.

Robins, L.N. and Przybeck, T.R. (1985). Age of onset of drug use as a factor in drug and other disorders. In C.L. Jones and R.L. Battjes, (Eds.). *Etiology of Drug Abuse: Implications for Prevention*. NIDA Research Monograph 56, National Institute on Drug Abuse, Rockville, MD., pp. 178–193.

Schuckit, M.A., Tipp, J.E., Smith, T.L., Shapiro, E., Hesselbrock, V.M., Bucholz, K.K., Reich, T., Nurnberger Jr., J.I. (1995). An evaluation of Type A and B alcoholics. *Addiction* 90(9), pp. 1189–1204.

Spence, S.H. (1997). Structure of anxiety symptoms among children: A confirmatory factor-analytic study. *Journal of Abnormal Psychology* 106(2), pp. 280–297.

Storr, C.L., Reboussin, B.A., and Anthony, J.C. (2004). Early childhood misbehavior and the estimated risk of becoming tobacco-dependent. *American Journal of Epidemiology* 160, pp. 126–130.

Substance Abuse and Mental Health Services Administration. (2003). *Results from the 2002 National Survey on Drug Use and Health: National Findings*. (Office of Applied Studies, NHSDA Series H-22, DHHS Publication No. SMA 03-3836). Rockville, MD.

Swendsen, J.D. and Merikangas, K.R. (2000). The comorbidity of depression and substance use disorders. *Clinical Psychology Review* 20, pp. 173–189.

Toomey, R. and Eaves, L. (1998). Co-occurrence of abuse of different drugs in men: the role of drug-specific and shared vulnerabilities. *Archives of General Psychiatry* 55, pp. 967–972.

Tsuang, M.T., Lyons, M.J., Meyer, J.M., Doyle, T., Eisen, S.A., Goldberg, J., True, W., Lin, N., Toomey, R., and Eaves, L. (1998). Co-occurrence of Abuse of Different Drugs in Men: The Role of Drug-Specific and Shared Vulnerabilities. *Archives of General Psychiatry* 55, pp. 967–972.

Tsuang, M.T., Lyons, M.J., Meyer, J.M., Doyle, T., Eisen, S.A., Goldberg, J., True, W., Lin, N., Warner, L.A., Kessler, R.C., Hughes, M., Anthony, J.C., and Nelson, C.B. (1995). Prevalence and correlates of drug use and dependence in the United States: results from the National Comorbidity Survey. *Archives of General Psychiatry* 52, 219–229.

Wagner, F.A. and Anthony, J.C. (2002). From first drug use to drug dependence: Developmental periods of risk for dependence upon marijuana, cocaine, and alcohol. *Neuropsychopharmacology* 26(4), pp. 479–488.

White, H.R., Xie, M., Thompson, W., Loeber, R., and Stouthamer-Loeber, M. (2001). Psychopathology as a predictor of adolescent drug use trajectories. *Psychology of Addictive Behaviors* 15, pp. 210–218.

World Health Organization. (1993). The *ICD-10 classification of mental and behavioural disorders: Clinical descriptions and diagnostic guidelines*. WHO, Geneva.

3

Studying the Natural History of Drug Use

Yih-Ing Hser, Douglas Longshore, Mary-Lynn Brecht and M. Douglas Anglin

YIH-ING HSER, DOUGLAS LONGSHORE, MARY-LYNN BRECHT AND M. DOUGLAS ANGLIN • UCLA Integrated Substance Abuse Programs, Neuropsychiatric Institute, University of California, Los Angeles

1. INTRODUCTION

To understand the process of drug use initiation, progression, addiction, cessation, and recovery, the importance of "natural history" or "drug use career" approaches has been increasingly emphasized (Anglin et al., 1997, 2001; Hser and Anglin, 1991; Hser et al., 1997; Maddux and Desmond, 1986; Sobell et al., 1993; Valillant, 1988, 1992). Findings in the United States have shown that patterns of lifetime drug use and related problems are extremely heterogeneous. Many people experiment with use and then desist, while a subset become frequent users, and only some of these become problematic or dependent users (Chen et al., 1997; Warner et al., 1995). For example, the National Drug Use and Health Survey (DUHS) shows that rates of use of illicit drugs other than marijuana are low (marijuana 39 percent, cocaine 14 percent, methamphetamine 5 percent, and heroin 2 percent). The small subset of serious users, once having initiated use, tends to continue and to accrue attendant problems until 'captured' in the criminal justice, health, or drug treatment system.

The only recurrent multi-city study assessing changes in adverse health effects is the Drug Abuse Warning Network (DAWN), by which hospitals and county coroners in selected cities report rates of drug use events or mentions in cases brought before them. DAWN data probably represent a broader range of users, from short-time users who have unexpected or mixed drug reactions to serious users who obtain an unexpectedly pure dose of their primary drug. Regarding the criminal justice system, the only multi-site national study of drug use among arrestees—and the only study to obtain urine for verification of self-report—was the Arrestee Drug Abuse Monitoring (ADAM) program, funded until 2004 by the National Institute of Justice. In the main however, only small, infrequent, and geographically limited epidemiological studies are conducted on the drug use of high social cost populations such as offenders, the mentally ill, the homeless, and so on. But it is in these populations that the majority of natural history studies have been conducted.

Altogether, research on the natural history of problematic drug use in the general population is scanty, and most knowledge about different aspects or stages of drug use careers is based, as noted, on more severe drug users whose health, mental health, and legal problems bring them into contact with the criminal justice system or social services. These are the populations least likely to be represented in national epidemiological surveys. For such 'system defined' groups, a consistent finding is the association of more serious drug use with other problematic behavior (emergency department visits, deaths reported to coroners, and so on), leading to the identification of drug users for study who have a certain history length and persisting pattern of use. Such samples are important since they represent socially high cost groups, but may not be representative of the natural history of less involved users.

A better understanding of the developmental and dynamic interplay between drug use overall, severe drug use, other problem behaviors, drug treatment, the criminal justice system, and other service systems is needed generally and will have important implications for improving practice and policy within and across these systems. Additionally, the natural history of drug use and its interplay with service systems also needs to be examined in specific demographic populations. In this chapter, we first provide our conceptual framework for study of the natural history of drug use as it occurs in the United States. Drawing from our own work and others, we describe patterns and correlates of initiation, progression, addiction, and cessation. The chapter then focuses on the natural history of drug use among individuals encountered in drug treatment, criminal justice, and mental health systems, followed by life-history differences with respect to gender and race/ethnicity. The chapter concludes with critical findings and suggests future research to improve the scientific knowledge on the natural history of drug use.

2.   CONCEPTUAL FRAMEWORK

In addition to research on the drug use career (Anglin et al., 2001; Hser et al., 1997; Nurco et al., 1975; 1994), which has established that addiction takes a chronic and relapsing course, we have drawn upon the "life course" concept in social psychology, the "illness career" concept in medical sociology, and the "criminal career" concept in criminology. Studies of the life course focus on the timing and consequences of change in social roles, e.g., marital status and occupation. Studies of the illness career have identified stages of illness beginning with problem recognition, health care utilization, primary compliance with caregiver advice, outcomes (e.g., recovery from or chronicity of illness), and secondary compliance (continuing in a long-term treatment regime) (Baltes et al., 1999; Pescosolido, 1991). Finally, we have drawn on research regarding the criminal career, i.e., "the longitudinal sequence of crimes committed by an individual offender" (Blumstein et al., 1986: 12). Criminal career researchers are engaged in mapping trajectories of offending, comparing these trajectories across different background characteristics of offenders, and measuring the interplay between criminal justice intervention and change in offending trajectories (Laub and Sampson, 2001; Piquero et al., 2003).

3.   DRUG USE PROGRESSION

The natural history of drug use can be considered in terms of drug use initiation and progression, persistent use, consequences, dependence and addiction, and cessation and recovery. Over the lifetime of a dependent user, some of these processes may repeat multiple times for the same or different substances. The key factors that influence drug use careers and associated consequences are of particular interest because they may have important implications for intervention development and policy decisions.

3.1. Drug Use Initiation and Progression

The work of Kandel and others has shown that among the general population, most drug use initiation occurs during the early teens, and almost no one initiates use of any illicit drug after age 29 (Chen and Kandel, 1995). While the causal significance of developmental stages remains unclear (Morral et al., 2002), studies have shown that adolescents are very unlikely to experiment with marijuana if they have not experimented previously with an alcoholic beverage or with cigarettes; similarly, very few try illicit drugs other than marijuana without prior use of marijuana (Brook et al., 1982; Donovan and Jessor, 1983; Kandel, 1975). As noted, most of these studies are primarily based on samples that included few serious drug users.

Other studies (Golub and Johnson, 1994; Mackesy-Amiti et al., 1997), based on samples of serious drug users, have found somewhat different sequences in drug use progression than those typically found in the general population. Golub and Johnson (1994) examined a sample of 994 serious drug users (e.g., those smoking crack or injecting heroin on a daily or more frequent basis) recruited in New York City in 1988–89. They found that alcohol use was not a typical prerequisite for progression to marijuana, but marijuana use nearly always preceded use of more serious substances such as cocaine, crack, and heroin. Their data also showed that among those serious substance abusers born in 1963 or later, marijuana appears to be more likely to precede any use of alcohol than the converse. The study results suggest the importance of considering birth cohort as a proxy for sociocultural context, since drug use developmental sequences may depend on the prevalence, availability, and accessibility of the various substances of the era and area. Thus, patterns of drug use initiation and progression may depend on sample characteristics, including regional histories of drug availability, overall level of drug involvement, mode of administration, concurrent behavioral or other problems, or birth cohorts of the sample under study (Johnson and Gerstein, 1998; Mackesy-Amiti et al., 1997; Warner et al., 1995).

Regardless of initiation sequences, however, age at initial use of alcohol, cigarettes, and illicit drugs has been shown to be a powerful predictor of subsequent consequences and dependence. Epidemiological and clinical studies suggest that adolescents who begin drug use at early ages typically use drugs more frequently, escalate to higher levels of use more quickly, and are more likely to persist in using (Anthony and Petronis, 1995; Yu and Williford, 1992).

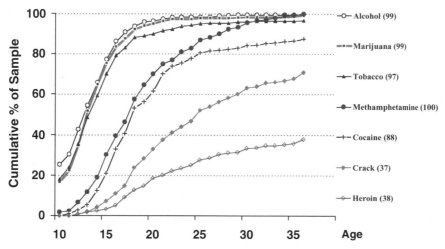

Figure 1. Age of initiation of seven drug types among a sample of methamphetamine users. [( )
indicates percent of sample ever reporting use]

3.2. Persistent Use

Because the proportions and numbers of serious drug users identified in general population studies are too low for rigorous scientific study, patterns of progression and persistence have been examined among populations in which higher proportions of individuals have progressed, or are likely to progress, to more serious levels of use. As one example to illustrate typical initiation patterns among those who ultimately become problematic users, Figure 1 shows the cumulative percent of a large Los Angeles sample of methamphetamine users arrayed by age of initiation for seven types of substances (Brecht et al., in submission). The so-called 'gateway' triad of alcohol, marijuana, and tobacco had been used by over 95 percent of the sample by age 20. Methamphetamine and cocaine use have similar patterns of initiation until about age 27, when methamphetamine use involved 100 percent of this sample and became the persisting drug of use. Crack and heroin use was reported by about 40 percent of the sample, and ages of initiation were more delayed and gradual than for other substances.

Long-term patterns of cocaine, methamphetamine, marijuana, and heroin use were studied by Hser and colleagues (1998) in a sample of approximately 1,800 drug users recruited from three high-risk settings (600 each from jails, hospital emergency rooms, and sexually transmitted diseases clinics) in Los Angeles County. A random subset of 566 drug users was followed over time to provide their natural history of drug use. Figure 2 shows patterns of at least weekly use of cocaine, methamphetamine, marijuana, and heroin by these individuals (Hser, 2002). There were distinct age-related trends for each drug. Marijuana and methamphetamine

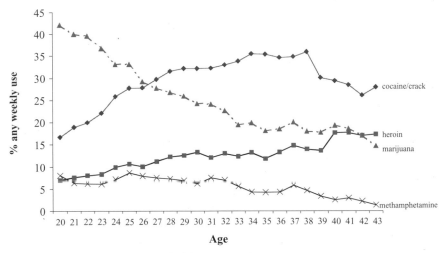

Figure 2. Self-reported weekly use of illicit drugs over time.

use showed linear declines as the cohort aged, although declines covered different age periods and occurred at different rates over time. Cocaine use increased from age 20 until the mid 30s and declined after the late 30s. Heroin use, on the other hand, increased with age. Thus, these findings clearly suggest that long-term trajectories of use among those who escalate to weekly use or more may differ by drug. Importantly, use peaks at different ages for such users, compared to users in the general population.

3.3. Consequences of Use

In a 33-year follow-up of a sample of 581 male narcotic addicts admitted to the California Civil Addict Program (a compulsory drug treatment program for opiate-dependent criminal offenders) from 1962 through 1964 (Hser et al., 2001), it was found that at the latest follow-up (1996/97), when the average age of this sample was 57 years, 284 were confirmed to be dead (48.9 percent), a much higher rate than in the general population of the same age. Death was most often caused by drug/alcohol overdose (21.6 percent), violence or accidents (19.5 percent), and medical conditions (chronic liver disease, 15.2 percent; cancer, 11.7 percent; and cardiovascular disease, 11.7 percent). Among the 242 addicts interviewed, about 40 percent reported past-year heroin use, and many reported current tobacco use (66.9 percent), daily drinking (22.1 percent), and drug use (e.g., past-year use of marijuana was reported by 35.5 percent, cocaine use by 19.4 percent, crack use by 10.3 percent, and methamphetamine use by 11.6 percent). The group also reported high rates of disability (43.8 percent), health problems (e.g., hepatitis, 41.7 percent), a variety of mental health problems, and criminal justice system involvement.

While mortality increased steadily and at a much higher rate than in the general population, opiate use patterns were remarkably stable; at average age 37, only 38 percent were opiate free at interview, a rate that increased to 41 percent by average age 48, and to 55.8 percent by average age 57. These slow rates of desistence suggest that cessation of opiate use is a very slow process and may not occur for those addicts who have not ceased use by their late 30s. Even among those abstinent for as long as 15 years, a quarter had relapsed in subsequent observations. Similarly, other research has shown that long-term cessation of heroin use is both slow and difficult process for many addicts and is preceded by repeated cycles of abstinence and relapse (Scott et al., 2003; Vaillant, 1992). In contrast, a long-term study of veterans who used heroin in Vietnam showed high remission rates once these veterans returned to home (Price et al., 2001), most often due to reduced stress, lack of drug availability, and return to civilian life with its social roles, benefits, and responsibilities. Another study of male alcohol abusers suggested that, unlike heroin use, relapse to alcohol use was typically rare after abstinence had been maintained for five years (Vaillant, 1996), suggesting that the inherent physiological differences between alcohol and heroin and the type of intervention and subsequent social support for recovery can produce very different outcomes.

In contrast to the heroin data reported above, Hser and colleagues have recently completed a 12-year follow-up study of 321 cocaine-dependent male veterans originally admitted in 1988–89 to their first treatment episode for cocaine dependence (2003a). Their cocaine use careers, from onset of use to treatment entry, averaged 11.5 years. Time-series analysis of severe cocaine use not only demonstrated dramatic reductions of cocaine use following treatment entry but also showed greater treatment effects by type of treatment utilized or longer treatment participation (Khalsa et al., 1993). The 12-year follow-up interviews, at average age 48, showed that although treatment entry at average age 36 produced a significant reduction in cocaine use, some 36 percent of those alive 12 years later reported cocaine/crack use in the prior year, and about 25 percent were positive for cocaine as evidenced by urinalysis (Hser et al., 2003a).

3.4. Cessation and Recovery

Only a few studies have examined cessation of illicit drug use among the general population (e.g., Chen and Kandel, 1998; Price et al., 2001; Vaillant, 1996). For example, some idea of desistance can be obtained from the DUHS by comparing ever use rates to past year rates, with the assumption that those reporting no use in the past year have discontinued their use of a particular drug.

By this rough guide, nearly half of those ever using marijuana had desisted and over 75 percent of cocaine users had desisted. By contrast, most studies on cessation or recovery from serious drug use are based on subjects selected from drug treatment programs for treatment evaluation purposes. Few studies have examined untreated users, either alone or as comparison groups for treated users. In such samples, desistence rates are, as noted in the prior section, less dramatic and frequently require intervention to produce.

3.4.1.   Cessation and Recovery in Treated Populations

Nearly all studies of drug treatment confirm the overall effectiveness of residential, outpatient, methadone maintenance, and other treatment modalities (Gerstein and Harwood, 1990; Hubbard et al., 1997; Simpson et al., 1999, 2002). However, the beneficial effect of any single treatment episode is often short-lived, and relapse to drug use is common (Hser et al., 1997; Nurco et al., 1994, Valliant, 1988). On the other hand, studies that focus on a single treatment episode typically ignore the effects of subsequent treatment. Among limited studies that have considered subsequent treatment, results generally suggest favorable outcomes among those reporting additional treatment(s). For example, Weisner and colleagues (2003) found that among those patients not abstinent at 6 months post-admission, treatment readmission was a significant predictor of abstinence at a five-year follow-up. This and other studies have demonstrated the beneficial impact of readmission for those not initially successful in treatment. Furthermore, for some patients, multiple treatment episodes are typical and may be necessary to achieve incremental improvements and eventual cessation (Anglin et al., 2001; Hser et al., 1997).

3.4.2.   Cessation and Recovery in Untreated Populations

Recovery can occur without treatment, and although the concept of "spontaneous recovery" is typically applied to less serious users, even severe drug users are capable of quitting as well (e.g., Cunningham et al., 1993). Unfortunately, rates of spontaneous recovery are not well documented; they come primarily from studies of alcohol users and qualitative studies on users of illicit drugs, and the evidence is neither consistent nor conclusive. Reviewing the literature on "spontaneous recovery" from alcohol abuse, Smart (1975) reported overall recovery rates varied across studies from 4 percent to 58 percent and yearly recovery rates since problem identification varied from less than 1 percent to 33 percent. This wide variation in reported rates can, to a great extent, be explained on methodological grounds (e.g., criteria of problematic use and definitions of remission). Some of the more optimistic conclusions on spontaneous recovery may be attributable to the study sample having only mild drug problems (cf. Lindstrom, 1992). Nevertheless, self-remitters studied by Sobell et al. (1992, 1993) and Klingemann (1991) were reported to have drinking or heroin use histories comparable in severity to various clinical samples. Thus, although the exact rates of self-remission from use of different drugs may vary and remain unclear, self-remission may occur even among people with consumption levels and duration of use similar to that of average clinical populations.

3.4.3.   Factors Influencing Recovery

Successful termination of problematic drug use results from a complex interactive process, including environmental influences, attitudinal changes, and reorientation of behavior. The exact nature of this interaction, the relative importance of contributing factors, and the context in which they occur are complicated and unclear. However, researchers have reported broad categories that seem applicable. Maddux and Desmond (1980) listed five conditions (relocation, religion, employment, probation/parole, and alcohol substitution) that probably facilitated three-year abstinence in 54 former heroin addicts. Waldorf et al. (1991) suggested six patterns of recovery from heroin use. For example, "situational change" was found to be the main path to recovery for addicts whose heroin use was situational. Working-class addicts living in communities with a high incidence of drug use and criminality reported the most difficulty trying to recover. Middle-class addicts with a greater array of resources either "matured out" by the simple process of aging and related life events (e.g., relocation, marriage, employment) or used other paths out of drug dependence. Maruna (2001) has documented similar patterns of cessation in the criminal career. The natural history approach captures the heterogeneity of recovery processes and provides the larger context in which to design, implement, and assess those policies and practices most likely to result in beneficial change.

4.   SPECIAL POPULATIONS

Although there are major commonalities in the natural history of many diverse types of substance users, it is important to describe patterns of the natural history for users of different demographic characteristics, and to assess how these factors affect the interplay between drug abuse, drug treatment, and other service systems. Below, we examine gender and racial/ethnic differences in the natural history of drug use and service system involvement.

4.1.   Gender Differences

Long-term patterns and correlates of drug use may differ by gender (Anglin et al., 1987a, 1987b; Chen and Kandel, 1998; Kandel, 2000; Yamaguchi and

Kandel, 1996). Some studies have shown that women tend to start using alcohol and other drugs at a later age than do men, but they enter into drug treatment after a briefer period of regular drug use (Anglin et al., 1987b) and may be more responsive to treatment (Hser et al., 2003b). While criminal justice involvement is a route to treatment for many users, women are less likely than men to be involved in crime and less often enter treatment under legal pressure (Grella et al., 2003). Several studies (e.g., Brady et al., 1993; Griffin et al., 1989) have reported more psychiatric disorders, particularly affective disorders (Wallen, 1992), among drug-using women than among drug-using men. Additionally, women users have more severe family and social problems (Brady et al., 1993; Grella et al., 2003; Hser et al., 2003b). Studies have also found that women are more likely to have substance using spouses and partners (Grella et al., 2003; Hser et al., 2003b) and that women's drug use is often influenced by their spouses or partners (e.g., Amaro and Hardy-Fanta, 1995). Women generally have lower levels of employment than do men and have primary responsibility for child rearing. They often lack the resources for transportation and childcare, which imposes barriers to their participation in treatment (Kline, 1996; Marsh et al., 2000). Thus, despite a shorter period of regular use before entering treatment, they often demonstrate more severe drug use and psychosocial disorders upon admission to treatment (Grella et al., 2003).

4.2. Racial/Ethnic Differences

Some studies have found racial/ethnic differences in drug use progression (Mackesy-Amiti et al., 1997; Yamaguchi and Kandel, 1996). Mackesy-Amiti et al. (1997) reported significant race/ethnicity effects for the typical progression (alcohol to marijuana to other drugs) versus atypical comparisons. For example, African Americans were less likely to use other illicit drugs before marijuana compared to non-African Americans. Hispanic addicts may begin using heroin at a younger age than other ethnicities (Trimble et al., 1987), yet time between first opiate use and progression to daily use was similar for Hispanics and Whites in Anglin et al. (1988). Typically, African Americans and Hispanics are over-represented in drug treatment in relation to their proportion of the population (NIDA, 1995), but racial/ethnic differences in treatment need have to be taken into account in studying treatment utilization. Among drug-using arrestees in Los Angeles, African Americans and Hispanics were less likely than Whites to think they needed treatment even though all were using drugs (mostly cocaine) on a daily basis (Longshore et al., 1993). Among persons who do enter treatment, outcomes may be less favorable for African Americans and Hispanics than for Whites (Prendergast et al., 1998; Trimble et al., 1987), although the evidence is not sufficient to support a firm conclusion (Brown and Alterman, 1992).

5. CONCLUDING COMMENTS

Drug use can escalate through myriad pathways to more severe levels. Once established, drug dependence frequently has a chronic, relapsing course lasting many years with multiple episodes of treatment and relapse, and stable cessation for many may be observable only in the long term. Accordingly, long-term strategies for curtailing drug use are unlikely to be optimally effective if based on studies with only short-term observations. Furthermore, drug users often come in contact with service systems other than drug treatment, and each system must be able to address not only the problem that brings clients to that system but their drug use and other problems as well. It is critical to take a longitudinal perspective in assessing drug use trajectories and interactions with a variety of service systems and to develop cross-system capabilities to serve the client and society.

Additional conceptual and methodological developments are needed to provide critical knowledge about patterns of drug use and cessation. Our 33-year follow-up study has shown that the eventual cessation of heroin use is a slow process that may not occur at all for some older addicts. However, it is not clear whether similar conclusions can be drawn about cocaine or methamphetamine users. Also, the similarities and differences that may exist in predictors of and pathways to cessation among users of these different drug types or among various special populations of drug users need further explication. Moreover, although many studies have shown that treatment generally reduces drug use and that rates of relapse and return to treatment are high, it is not known how drug use characteristics (e.g., consequences, severity, and chronicity) and treatment characteristics (e.g., type, intensity, and frequency) interact to produce the desired outcomes. Finally, studying predictors and correlates of drug use cessation, relapse, and episodic recovery is important in understanding the process of sustained recovery from dependence. Findings from such studies have practical implications for designing more effective intervention strategies, not only for those who seek formal treatment but also for the many drug-dependent users who do not. The improved scientific understanding of long-term drug use patterns and clinical/services research will expand our ability to develop effective longer-term clinical and policy strategies.

REFERENCES

Amaro, H. and Hardy-Fanta, C. (1995). Gender relations in addiction and recovery. *Journal of Psychoactive Drugs* 27, pp. 325–337.

Anglin, M. D., Booth, M. W., Ryan, T. M. and Hser, Y. (1988). Ethnic differences in narcotics addiction. II. Chicano and Anglo Addiction Career Patterns. *International Journal of the Addictions* 23(10), pp. 1011–1027.

Anglin, M. D., Hser, Y.-I. and Booth, M. W. (1987a). Sex differences in addict careers. 4. Treatment. *American Journal of Drug and Alcohol Abuse* 13(3), pp. 253–280.

Anglin, M. D., Hser, Y.-I. and Grella, C. E. (1997). Drug addiction and treatment careers among clients in DATOS. *Psychology of Addictive Behaviors* 11(4), pp. 308–323.

Anglin, M. D., Hser, Y.-I., Grella, C. E., Longshore, D. and Prendergast, M. L. (2001). Drug treatment careers: Conceptual overview and clinical, research, and policy applications. In: F. M. Tims, C. G. Leukefeld, and J. J. Platt (Eds.), *Relapse and recovery in addictions* (pp.18–39). Yale University Press, New Haven and London.

Anglin, M. D., Hser, Y.-I. and McGlothlin, W. H. (1987b). Sex differences in addict careers. 2. Becoming addicted. *American Journal of Drug and Alcohol Abuse* 13(1–2), pp. 59–71.

Anthony, J. C. and Petronis, K. R. (1995). Early-onset drug use and risk of later drug problems. *Drug and Alcohol Dependence* 40(1), pp. 9–15.

Baltes, P. V., Staudinger, U. M. and Lindenberger, U. (1999). Lifespan psychology: Theory and application to intellectual functioning. *Annual Review of Psychology* 50, pp. 471–507.

Blumstein, A., Cohen J, Roth, J. A. and Visher, C. A. (1986). (Eds.), *Criminal careers and career criminal. Volumes 1 and 2.* National Academy Press, Washington, D.C.

Brady, K. T., Grice, D. E., Dustan, L., and Randall, C. (1993). Gender differences in substance use disorders. *American Journal of Psychiatry* 150, pp. 1707–1711.

Brook, J. S., Whiteman, M., and Gordon, A. S. (1982). Qualitative and quantitative aspects of adolescent drug use: interplay of personality, family, and peer correlates. *Psychological Reports* 51(3), pp. 1151–1163.

Brown L. S, and Alterman A. (1992). African Americans. In: J. H. Lowinson, P. Ruiz, R. B. Millman, and J. G. Langrod (Eds.), *Substance abuse: A comprehensive textbook* (pp. 861–867). Williams and Wilkins, Baltimore, Maryland.

Chen, K., and Kandel, D. B. (1995). The natural history of drug use from adolescence to the mid-thirties in a general population sample. *American Journal of Public Health* 85(1), pp. 41–47.

Chen, K., and Kandel, D. B. (1998). Predictors of cessation of marijuana use: An event history analysis. *Drug and Alcohol Dependence* 50(2), pp.109–121.

Chen, K., Kandel, D. B., and Davies, M. (1997). Relationships between frequency and quantity of marijuana use and last year proxy dependence among adolescents and adults in the United States. *Drug and Alcohol Dependence* 46(1–2), pp. 53–67.

Clark, D. B., Kirisci, L., and Tarter, R. E. (1998). Adolescent versus adult onset and the development of substance use disorders in males. *Drug and Alcohol Dependence* 49(2), pp. 115–121.

Cunningham, J. A., Sobell, L. C., Sobell, M. B., Agrawal, S., and Toneatto, T. (1993). Barriers to treatment: Why alcohol and drug abusers delay or never seek treatment. *Addictive Behaviors* 18, pp. 347–353.

Donovan, J. E., and Jessor, R. (1983). Problem drinking and the dimension of involvement with drugs: A guttman scalogram analysis of adolescent drug use. *American Journal of Public Health* 73, pp. 543–552.

Gerstein, D. R. E., and Harwood, H. J. E. (1990). *Treating drug problems: A study of the evolution, effectiveness, and financing of public and private drug treatment systems.* National Academy of Sciences, Institute of Medicine. Division of Health Care Services, Committee for the Substance Abuse Coverage Study. National Academy Press, Washington, D.C.

Golub, A., Johnson, B. D. (1994). The shifting importance of alcohol and marijuana as gateway substances among serious drug abusers. *Journal of Studies on Alcohol,* 55(5), 607–614.

Grella, C. E., Scott, C. K., Foss, M. A., Joshi, V., and Hser, Y.-I. (2003). Gender differences in drug treatment outcomes among participants in the Chicago Target Cities Study. *Evaluation and Program Planning* 26(30), pp. 297–310.

Griffin, M. L., Weiss, R. D., Mirin, S. M., and Lange, U. (1989). A comparison of male and female cocaine abusers. *Archives of General Psychiatry* 46(2), pp. 122–126.

Hser, Y.-I. (2002). *Drug use careers: Recovery and mortality. OAS Monograph: The future impact of substance use by older persons: Approaches to estimation and the implications for the treatment system.* Office of Applied Study, SAMHSA, Rockville, Maryland.

Hser, Y.-I., and Anglin, M. D. (1991). Cost-effectiveness of drug abuse treatment: Relevant issues and alternative longitudinal modeling approaches. *NIDA Research Monograph* 113, pp. 67–93.

Hser, Y.-I., Anglin, M. D., Grella, C., Longshore, D., and Prendergast, M. (1997). Drug treatment careers: A conceptual framework and existing research findings. *Journal of Substance Abuse Treatment* 14(6), pp. 543–558.

Hser, Y.-I., Boles, S. M., Stark, M. E., Paredes, M., Huang, Y., Rawson, R., and Anglin, M. D. (2003, June). *A 12 –year follow-up of a cocaine-dependent sample.* Poster presented at the College on Problems of Drug Dependence, 65th Annual Scientific Meeting, San Juan, Puerto Rico.

Hser, Y.-I., Boyle, K., and Anglin, M. D. (1998). Drug use and correlates among sexually transmitted disease patients, emergency room patients, and arrestees. *Journal of Drug Issues* 28(2), pp. 437–454.

Hser, Y.-I., Hoffman, V., Grella, C.E., and Anglin, M.D. (2001). A 33-year follow-up of narcotics addicts. *Archives of General Psychiatry* 58, pp. 503–508.

Hser, Y.-I., Huang, Y, Teruya, C., and Anglin, M. D. (2003a). Gender differences in drug abuse treatment outcomes and correlates. *Drug and Alcohol Dependence* 72, pp. 255–264.

Hubbard, R. L., Craddock, S. G., Flynn, P. M., Anderson, J. and Etheridge, R. (1997). Overview of 1-year follow-up outcomes in the Drug Abuse Treatment Outcome Study (DATOS). *Psychology of Addictive Behaviors* 11(4), pp. 261–278.

Johnson, R. A., and Gerstein, D. R. (1998). Initiation of use of alcohol, cigarettes, marijuana, cocaine, and other substances in US birth cohorts since 1919. *American Journal of Public Health* 88(1), pp. 27–33.

Kandel, D. (1975). Stages in adolescent involvement in drug use. *Science* 190(4217), pp. 912–914.

Kandel, D. B. (2000). Gender differences in the epidemiology of substance dependence in the United States. In E. Frank (Ed.), *Gender and its effects on psychopathology* (pp. 231–252). American Psychiatric Press, Washington, D.C.

Khalsa, M. E., Paredes, A., and Anglin, M. D. (1993). Cocaine dependence: behavioral dimensions and patterns of progression. *American Journal on Addictions* 2, pp. 330–345.

Kline, A. (1996). Pathways into drug user treatment: The influence of gender and racial/ethnic identity. *Substance Use and Misuse* 31(3), pp. 323–342.

Klingemann, H. K. (1991). The motivation for change from problem alcohol and heroin use. *British Journal of Addiction* 86(6), pp. 727–744.

Laub, J. H., and Sampson, R. J. (2001). Understanding desistance from crime. In M. Tonry (Ed.), *Crime and justice: A review of research* (pp. 2–69). The University of Chicago Press, Chicago.

Leshner, A. I. (1999). Science-based views of drug addiction and its treatment. *Journal of the American Medical Association* 282(14), pp. 1314–1316.

Lindström, L. (1992). *Managing alcoholism.* Oxford University Press, Oxford.

Longshore, D., Hsieh, S., and Anglin, M. D. (1993). Ethnic and gender differences in drug users' perceived need for treatment. *International Journal of the Addictions* 28(6), pp. 539–558.

Mackesy-Amiti, M. E., Fendrich, M., and Goldstein, P. J. (1997). Sequence of drug use among serious drug users: typical vs atypical progression. *Drug and Alcohol Dependence* 45(3), pp. 185–196.

Maddux, J. F., and Desmond, D. P. (1980). New light on the maturing hypothesis in opioid dependence. *Bulletin on Narcotics* 32, pp. 15–25.

Maddux, J. F., and Desmond, D. P. (1986). Relapse and recovery in substance abuse careers. In F. M. Tims, and C. G. Leukefeld (Eds.), *Research Analysis and Utilization System: Relapse and Recovery in Drug Abuse.* National Institute on Drug Abuse Monograph 72, National Institute on Drug Abuse, Rockville, Maryland.

Marsh, J. C., D'Aunno, T. A., and Smith, B. D. (2000). Increasing access and providing social services to improve drug abuse treatment for women with children. *Addiction* 95(8), pp. 1237–1247.

Maruna, S. (2001). *Making Good*. American Psychological Association, Washington, D.C.

Morral, A. R., McCaffrey, D. F., and Paddock, S. M. (2002). Reassessing the marijuana gateway effect. *Addiction* 97(12), pp. 1493–1504.

National Institute on Drug Abuse (1995). *Drug use among racial/ethnic minorities*. NIH publication 95-3888. Department of Health and Human Services, Rockville, Maryland.

Nurco, D. N., Balter, M. B., and Kinlock, T. (1994). Vulnerability to narcotic addiction: Preliminary findings. *Journal of Drug Issues* 24(1–2), pp. 293–314.

Nurco, D. N., Bonito, A. J., Lerner, M. and Balter, M. B. (1975). Studying addicts over time: Methodology and Preliminary Findings. *American Journal of Drug and Alcohol Abuse* 2 (2), pp. 183–196.

Pescosolido, B.A. (1991). Illness careers and network ties: A conceptual model of utilization of compliance. *Advances in Medical Sociology* 2, pp. 161–184.

Piquero, A. R., Farrington, D. P., and Blumstein, A. (2003). Criminal career paradigm. In M. Tonry (Ed.), *Crime and Justice: Vol. 130* (pp. 359–506). University of Chicago Press, Chicago.

Price, R. K., Risk, N. K., and Spitznagel, E. L. (2001). Remission from drug abuse over a 25-year period: Patterns of remission and treatment use. *American Journal of Public Health* 91(7), pp. 1107–1013.

Scott, C.K., Foss, M.A., and Dennis M.L. (2003a). Factors influencing initial and longer-term responses to substance abuse treatment: A path analysis. *Evaluation and Program Planning* 26,pp. 287–296.

Simpson, D. D., Joe, G. W., and Broome, K. M. (2002). A national 5-year follow-up of treatment outcomes for cocaine dependence. *Archives of General Psychiatry* 59, pp. 538–544.

Simpson, D. D., Joe, G. W., Fletcher, B. W., Hubbard, R. L., and Anglin, M. D. (1999). A national evaluation of treatment outcomes for cocaine dependence. *Archives of General Psychiatry* 56(6), pp. 507–514.

Smart, R. G. (1975). Spontaneous recovery in alcoholics: A review and analysis of the available research. *Drug and Alcohol Dependence* 1, pp. 277–285.

Sobell, L. C., Cunningham, J. A., Sobell, M. B., and Toneatto, T. (1993). A life span perspective on natural recovery (self-change) from alcohol problems. In: J. S. Baer, G. A. Marlatt, and R. J. McMahon (Eds.), *Addictive behaviors across the life span: Prevention, treatment and policy issues* (pp. 35–66). Sage, Newbury Park, CA.

Sobell, L. C., Sobell, M. B., and Toneatto, T. (1992). Recovery from alcohol problems without treatment. N. Heather, W. R. Miller, and J. Greeley (Eds.), *Self-control and the addictive behaviors* (pp. 198–242). Maxwell MacMillan, New York.

Turner, W. M., Cutter, H. S., Worobec, T. G., O'Farrell, T. J., Bayog, R. D., and Tsuang, M. T. (1993). Family history models of alcoholism: age of onset, consequences and dependence. *Journal of Studies on Alcohol* 54(2), pp. 164–171.

Trimble, J. E, Padilla, A. M. and Bell, C. S. (1987). *Drug abuse among ethnic minorities*. Department of Health and Human Services, Rockville, Maryland.

Vaillant, G. E. (1988). What can long-term follow-up teach us about relapse and prevention of relapse in addiction? *British Journal of Addiction* 83(10), pp. 1147–1157.

Vaillant, G. E. (1992). Is there a natural history of addiction? In C. P. O'Brien and J. H. Jaffe (Eds.), *Addictive States*. Raven Press, New York.

Vaillant, G. E. (1996). A long-term follow-up of male alcohol abuse. *Archives of General Psychiatry* 53, pp. 243–249.

Waldorf, D., Reinarman, C. and Murphy, S. (1991). *Cocaine Changes*. Temple University Press, Philadelphia.

Wallen, J. (1992). A comparison of male and female clients in substance abuse treatment. *Journal of Substance Abuse Treatment* 9(3), pp. 243–248.

Warner, L. A., Kessler, R. C., Hughes, M., Anthony, J. C. and Nelson, C. B. (1995). Prevalence and correlates of drug use and dependence in the United States. Results from the National Comorbidity Survey. *Archives of General Psychiatry* 52(3), pp. 219–229.

Weisner, C., Ray, G. T., Mertens, J., Satre, D. and Moore, C. (2003). Short-term alcohol and drug treatment outcomes predict long-term outcome. *Drug and Alcohol Dependence* 70(3), pp. 81–294.

Yamaguchi, K. and Kandel, D. B. (1996). Parametric event sequence analysis: An application to an analysis of gender and racial/ethnic differences in patterns of drug-use progression. *Journal of the American Statistical Association* 91(436), pp. 1388–1399.

Yu, J. and Williford, W. R. (1992). The age of alcohol onset and alcohol, cigarette, and marijuana use patterns: an analysis of drug use progression of young adults in New York state. *International Journal of the Addictions* 27(11), pp. 1313–1323.

4

Health, Social, and Psychological Consequences of Drug Use and Abuse

Michael D. Newcomb and Thomas Locke

MICHAEL D. NEWCOMB • University of Southern California
THOMAS LOCKE • University of California, Los Angeles

1. INTRODUCTION

Several epidemiological researchers have begun a theoretical integration of the rather rich drug use and abuse etiology literature and the far less developed and somewhat paltry drug use and abuse consequences research findings. This integration has numerous advantages as well as theoretical and methodological challenges (Newcomb, 2004). It is beyond this chapter to delineate this synergy in much detail. However, the central focus of this approach is to consider drug use and abuse as mediators. A mediator is operationalized as a "generative mechanism through which the focal independent variable is able to influence the dependent variable of interest" (Baron and Kenny, 1986, P. 1173). Therefore, mediators (drug use and abuse) are predicted by various risk and protective factors. Also, they themselves are the predictors of later consequences and outcomes.

The underlying assumptions of drug use prevention programs are that their interventions will somehow reduce or eliminate the presumed adverse consequences related to drug use. Because of the intense focus on preventing drug use, funding and support for studies of the consequences of drug use has been minimal. By preventing drug use and abuse the wide spread adverse and devastating consequences of drug use both proximally (immediately) and distally (later in life) will also be prevented. Most in the field believe that drug abuse has many assumed catastrophic consequences for the individual, their friends and family, and society. Some supportive evidence exists. For instance, drug use during adolescence appears to have both short-term and long-term effects on cognitive and brain functioning (Brown et al., 2000; White, 2004). Yet there is a dearth of scientific evidence to firmly establish what these adverse consequences are, what mechanisms are involved, and how they might present in various psychosocial domains.

As a result, consequence components and related theoretical aspects of prevention programs may be targeting too many domains, omitting others, and thereby may be mis-directed. Accurate and realistic information on the consequences of drug ingestion is important not only for prevention and for treatment programming but also for making policy addressing the health, social and psychological needs of drug abusers.

Although not typically conceived of as such, the *Diagnostic and Statistical Manual of Mental Disorders—4th Edition* (American Psychiatric Association, 1994) diagnostic criteria are largely based on consequences of drug ingestion or the pursuit of the substance. Examples of these include, "important social, occupational, or recreational activities are given up or reduced because of substance use" and "the substance use is continued despite knowledge of having a persistent or recurrent physical or psychological problem that is likely to be caused or exacerbated by the substance . . . " (p. 181). Syndromes associated with substance intoxication and with withdrawal are also described. However, drug use that does not reach the level of severe psychosocial impairment is not necessarily considered. Therefore, there is an implication that drug use that does not meet the DSM-IV criteria for substance-use disorders is acceptable and does not promote adverse consequences.

Overall, research that focuses on drug using populations has shown that the consequences of drug use affect many areas of an individual's life. Some of the noted biological consequences include various areas such as HIV transmission and acquisition, neuro-cognitive impairment, heart disease, intergenerational transmission of biological predisposition, mortality/morbidity, and health-service utilization. Psychological consequences can include many domains such as mood disorders, anxiety, other psychiatric disorders, and disruption in adaptive coping mechanisms, attachment disruption, anger management, and suicidal ideation. Social domains that are often implicated include marital and relationship satisfaction, employment stability and satisfaction, educational attainment, legal issues/criminal behavior, parenting, and social support. However, the study of both long- and short-term consequences is challenged, primarily as assignment of the attribution of the impact of drug using behaviors is not always clear. There are two components to the assignment of attribution. The first relates to whether the consequences of drug use are direct, indirect or the result of the drug mediating or moderating of another process that is taking place. The second relates to the methodological difficulties of establishing causation.

2. DEFINING THE ROLE OF DRUG USE

Drug use consequences can be thought of as relating to three main processes: direct, indirect, and mediating/moderating effects. Direct effects vary across different developmental periods and are related to the specific influence of a drug on later outcome biopsychosocial functioning. Indirect effects are related to the influence of another person's drug use (parents, peers, partners) on the individual's life (e.g., psychological distress due to a partner's drug use). Indirect effects emphasize the importance of a systemic or holistic point of view. Finally, drug use can serve as a factor that alters other processes that may already be in play. Studying drug use as a moderator investigates how it "affects the relationship between two variables, so that the nature of the impact of the predictor on the criterion varies according to the level or value of the moderator (also see Saunders, 1956; Zedeck, 1971). *Further*, a moderator interacts with a predictor variable in such a way as to have an impact on the level of a dependent variable" (Holmbeck, 1997, p. 600). This can be represented in questions such as . . . Can drug use exacerbate the effects of a poor upbringing? As a mediator, drug use is viewed as a "generative mechanism through which the focal independent variable is able to influence the dependent variable of interest" (Baron and Kenny, 1986, P. 1173). This process can be represented in questions such as . . . Does drug use influence the relationship between early experience and later development?

Appropriate, new, and innovative statistical methods can help estimate unique variance due to drug use/abuse when not accounted for by other competing independent variables. For instance, structural equation modeling allows for the simultaneous estimation of multiple independent variables with an approximation of variance explained and unexplained by each on given outcome variables. This is a way to maximize causal inference and try to account for or estimate the influence the specific and unique influence of drug use on different aspects of later psychosocial functioning.

3.   METHODOLOGICAL ISSUES

Numerous methodological issues exist that make consequence research challenging. These issues are critical to consider in testing for and establishing the consequences of drug use. These include difficulty with operational definitions, research design, and the samples used.

3.1.   Criteria of Association

Criteria to establish a direct relationship between drug use and "consequences" include: 1) a process, issue, or psychosocial outcome whose existing state or pre-morbid condition changes because of drug use; 2) the change in these outcomes is subsequent to drug use; 3) these outcomes would not change in the same way without the use of drug(s) (Newcomb, 1994); and 4) these consequences are not due to factors other than drug use. Further, it is important to conceptualize drug use consequences as being immediate or short-term, intermediate, and long-term (Newcomb, 1997).

3.1.1.   Short-Term Consequences

Short-term consequences of drug use are relatively easy to establish through true experimental designs. For instance, establishing the direct physiological affect of a substance such as alcohol on reaction time can be accomplished with this method. Other more innovative approaches have also been developed such as the balanced placebo design (Marlatt et al., 1988). In this design, the expectancy effects of using a drug can be separated from the true pharmacological effects of the drug. Other more naturally occurring tragic short-term consequences include overdoses, car crashes due to alcohol or other drugs, and increased aggression and confrontational acts.

3.1.2.   Long-Term Consequences

Long-term drug use consequences are far more difficult to establish than are those that are considered short-term. The primary reason for this is that true experimental control over the types of drugs used and the duration of their use is not possible. Therefore, it is difficult to establish how such use influences functioning later in life. For instance, it is not ethical to randomly assign one group of sixth graders to smoke one joint of marijuana every day and another matched group of sixth graders to never smoke marijuana to determine how the two groups differ in their level of functioning later in life. Therefore the only alternative is to follow the naturally unfolding development of individuals over time and repeatedly assess their drug use and their evolving biopsychosocial maturation.

In order to establish causal inferences for long-term drug use consequences four assumptions must be met. First, there must be a reliable association between drug use and the outcome or consequence. Second, drug use must temporally precede the consequence. Third, the drug use must make a change in the consequence. Using both baseline and outcome measures of the consequence to show that drug use contributes unique variance above and beyond the specific stability effect. Finally, it is important to show that these relationships are not spurious and due to third-variable factors. This final assumption is not always possible to satisfy, and represents an inherent limitation in consequence research. However, using complex multivariate models that explicitly include alternate predictors of the outcomes is a powerful, but still not definite, approach to use to determine the plausible causal inferences of drug use on later consequences.

3.2.   Additional Methodological Issues

Several additional points are important to mention as a backdrop for this discussion. First, it is important to consider that consequences may be different for quantity of drug use versus frequency of drug use (Stein et al., 1988). Second, short-term consequences of drug use may have their own unique long-term effects, which may or may not be the same long-term consequences of the use of the drug alone. Third, since the use of one or more substances is relatively common, using a statistical method that can tease-out the specific effects of the use of a particular substance from the general effect of polydrug use is important (Newcomb, 1994). Fourth, consequences of substance use result from cumulative use, may respond to a change (increase or decrease) in substance use, or may occur once a particular threshold of use is crossed. Finally, consequences of drug use are different at different ages (Newcomb and Jack, 1995). For instance, alcohol use as a teenager may predict educational drop-out but stronger social skills and positive self concept (Newcomb and Bentler, 1988), whereas as a young adult it may predict poor parenting skills later in life (Locke and Newcomb, 2004).

In addition to methodological limitations regarding research design, another consideration relates to the nature of the samples used in consequence research. Much of existing research uses treatment or clinical samples. People within these samples typically have more serious problems with substances, and may very well have additional psychosocial conditions which may impair their functioning.

Applying information obtained from these samples to the community at large has inherent problems.

4. SELECTIVE REVIEW OF DRUG USE CONSEQUENCES

Many short-term and long-term consequences of drug use have been investigated. This section reviews and categorizes findings in three broad areas, health consequences, psychological consequences, and social consequences. Since these domains encompass such a wide range of topics and human behaviors, this review is not exhaustive. Rather, specific areas within each domain are selectively reviewed. The review on health consequences includes HIV-sexual risk behaviors, health-service utilization, and morbidity/mortality statistics. The section on psychological consequences focuses on suicidality, depression, anxiety, and psychosis. The section on social consequences is focused on interpersonal relationships. Specifically, antisocial behavior (theft and violent crime), interpersonal relationships (marital satisfaction, divorce, parenting), and workplace involvement (absenteeism, job satisfaction and stability) will be reviewed. Since both short-term and long-term consequences are important to consider, both cross-sectional and prospective studies are included in the following review.

4.1. Health

Various short-term health consequences associated with drug use have been established (over-doses, aggression, accidents). Long-term consequences have been more difficult to adequately test as the physiological mechanisms are more difficult to determine. The use of cigarettes is associated with cancer, emphysema, and heart disease. Cigarette smoking is responsible for over 400,000 deaths per year. Alcohol use is responsible for over 400,000 alcohol-related traffic crash deaths per year and over 25,000 people die from cirrhosis of the liver (National Institute on Alcohol Abuse and Alcoholism, 2004). Illicit drug use is associated with many health consequences including death (suicide, homicide, motor-vehicle injury) HIV infection, pneumonia, violence, and hepatitis. Overall, it is estimated that illicit drug use resulted in approximately 17,000 deaths in 2000 (Mokdad et al., 2004).

Drug abuse is often an important determinant or correlate of sexual risk behaviors (Tapert et al., 2001; Testa and Collins, 1997). Drugs are used to enhance the sexual experience or the engagement in sexual behaviors helps to support the costs of drugs. Drug use has consistently been found to significantly increase sexual and other risk behaviors in many diverse populations. For instance, in a large community-based sample of male Latinos, Locke et al., (in press) found that drug use predicted more partners, more pregnancies, and more HIV testing. Further, another study (Newcomb et al., 2003) found that drug use mediated the influence of physical and emotional abuse on sexual risk behaviors in a large community sample of Latinas. Overall, behavior associated with drug abuse is now the single largest factor in the spread of HIV infection in the United States. In the United States, an estimated one-third of HIV/AIDS cases are related to injecting drug use. The use of drugs injected or not, can affect decision making—particularly about engaging in unsafe sex—that can endanger one's health and the health of others (National Institute on Drug Abuse, 2003).

Ellickson et al., (2004) studied the adult behavioral, socioeconomic, and health outcomes of adolescent and young adult marijuana users in a large prospective community sample. They identified several groups of individuals: those who abstained from marijuana use, early high users, stable light users, steady increasers, and occasional light users. Growth mixture analysis was conducted on six-waves of data on marijuana users collected over a 10-year period. After controlling for gender, race-ethnicity, household composition, and parental education, they found that the early high users had significantly poorer overall health than all other groups. Further, they had significantly lower earnings and lower educational attainment than all but the stable light users. Abstainers outperformed all other groups by age 29 in the domains of educational achievement, overall health, and life satisfaction.

Those who abuse drugs often have higher levels of health service utilization than those who do not (Newcomb and Bentler, 1987). Palepu et al., (2003) examined emergency department utilization in a longitudinal study of HIV-infected persons with a history of alcohol problems. They found that substance abuse treatment was significantly related to decreased emergency room visits. However, the effect may be different for different substances, and may not be entirely linear. Cherpitel (2003) examined health service utilization in the US using two large national surveys conducted in 1995 and 2000. It was found that those reporting any health services utilization were less likely to report heavy drinking, two or more alcohol problems, and symptoms of alcohol dependence. Heavy or problem drinking was not predictive of health services utilization. After controlling for demographic characteristics and health insurance coverage, illicit drug users were almost twice as likely compared with nonusers, to report ER utilization, and one and a half times more likely to report primary care utilization in the 2000 survey, even though drug use was not significantly predictive of health services utilization in 1995.

4.2. Mental Health

A few longitudinal studies have examined the mental health consequences of drug use in general community populations, and varied findings have emerged (e.g.,

Kandel et al., 1986; Newcomb and Bentler, 1987; 1988). Some have reported causal relationships between drug use and deteriorated emotional health (e.g., Dackis and Gold, 1983; Newcomb and Bentler, 1987; 1988). Vaillant's (1995, 1993) highly cited, yet controversial study of male college students yields some interesting findings. He found that those who abused alcohol were five times more likely to report being severely depressed than those who did not. Vaillant's assertion that alcoholism is rarely the result of depression, but it is often a major causative factor, supports other views in the literature (e.g., Schuckitt, 1986), but it is disconcerting that he based this on such a small sample (N = 14). Further, while this is considered a community study, it is of males from Harvard University and therefore is not representative of the college-aged population. Overall, though accepted as common knowledge, evidence for causal relationships between early drug use and later deficits in emotional development is "hard to verify scientifically" (Newcomb and Bentler, 1988, p. 64). For example, adequate controls for preexisting conditions and important confounds may not have been made.

Another longitudinal prospective study found a reciprocal effect between substance involvement and psychological distress (dysphoria and suicidal ideation), with substance use serving as both a predictor and outcome of psychological distress. Specifically, Newcomb et al., (1999) found that as an individual progressed through adulthood, psychological functioning was impaired by substance problems experienced four years earlier. In addition, they found that substance involvement was influenced by earlier psychological distress. Christoffersen et al., (2003) also found that suicide risk was associated with prior drug addiction in a prospective register-based study of Danish children.

Newcomb et al., (1993) used prospective data from a community sample of 487 participants who were assessed 4 times over 12 years, beginning when they were young adolescents. They found that teenage polydrug use had few direct or unique effects on adult mental health, whereas increased polydrug use exacerbated later psychoticism, suicide ideation, and other indicators of emotional distress. Specific drug use in adolescence and changes in usage patterns into young adulthood predicted later psychopathology. Pencer and Addington (2003) also found that substance use was related to higher positive psychotic symptoms.

Locke and Newcomb (2001) found several reciprocal relationships between alcohol use and dysphoria for both men and women over a 16-year period from adolescence to adulthood. For women, dysphoria during young adulthood had serious consequences, leading to alcohol-related problems and use of alcohol at work during adulthood. Also, alcohol involvement in young adulthood led to specific aspects of dysphoria in adulthood. For men, alcohol involvement during late adolescence led to depression as measured by the CES-D in adulthood, and depression scale scores in late adolescence led to alcohol involvement in adulthood. Also, suicidal ideation during late adolescence predicted use of alcohol at work in adulthood.

In a longitudinal study of adolescents, Shedler and Block (1990) found that those who had engaged in some drug experimentation were the best-adjusted of all participants. Those who frequently used drugs were maladjusted, and displayed interpersonal alienation, poor impulse control, and manifest emotional distress. If an adolescent had not experimented with any drug by age 18, they were relatively anxious, emotionally constricted, and lacking in social skills. Further, several studies have reported apparently positive effects from moderate alcohol use, including greater positive affect, stress reduction, and limited improvements in cognitive performance (Baum-Baicker, 1985; Kandel et al., 1986; Newcomb and Bentler, 1987, 1988; Newcomb et al., 1986).

4.3. Antisocial Behavior

Although there is a clear correlation between drug use and criminality, several problems contribute to uncertainty as to how they are causally related in the general population. First, a focus on only clinical samples (e.g., Hanlon et al., 1990), adults in the criminal justice system (Harrison, 1992; Innes and Greenfeld, 1990), or adolescent samples (e.g., Apospori et al., 1995) limits the generalizability of the results to community samples of adults. Nevertheless, the association between drug abuse and criminal behavior and delinquency in the general population has been examined (e.g., Kaplan, 1995). Second, cross-sectional data prohibit the elucidation of the causal relation between drug abuse and criminal behavior. Third, many previous studies have examined specific types of drug use and not polydrug use, which might more likely be related to criminal behavior as it suggests a more deviant lifestyle of drug abuse. Therefore, whether drug problems precede criminality or criminal behaviors precede drug problems continues to be debated (Kaplan and Damphousse, 1995). Finally, the potential influence of other contributing or explanatory factors, such as social support and social conformity, have received little attention.

Brook et al. (2003) tested associations between marijuana use and several domains of behavior 2 years later in a community-based sample of 1,151 male and 1,075 female Colombian adolescents. Findings suggest that time 1 adolescent marijuana use was associated with increased risks for time 2 adolescent difficulty in a variety of domains including violent experiences. The findings suggest that early adolescent marijuana use is associated with an increase in problem behavior during later adolescence.

Newcomb et al. (2001) used prospective data to test the associations between drug abuse and crime in a community sample of 470 adults. Polydrug problems in early adulthood predicted both criminal behavior and polydrug problems in adulthood. Consequences of drug problems as a young adult included arrests and convictions for drug-related offenses, property damage, and driving under the influence of other drugs. Predictors of later polydrug problems included thefts, driving under the influence of alcohol and other drugs, arrests and convictions for drug-related offenses, and a lack of support for drug problems. Theoretical implications of these findings are discussed.

4.4. Interpersonal Relationships

The two key consequence areas relative to interpersonal relationships that have been studies are parenting practices and workplace behaviors.

4.4.1. Impact on Adult Parenting Practices

"The presence of substance abuse in an adult may or may not be an indicator that he or she is a dysfunctional parent" (Mayes, 1995 p. 101). Most work involving the influence of drug use on parenting looks at treatment or clinical samples. A few community studies have found associations between drug use and poor parenting. Newcomb and Loeb (1999) found poor parenting to be associated with a cluster of adult deviant behaviors that included polydrug problems and crime. Overall, it appears that drug-using parents are more likely to live unconventional lifestyles and endorse nonconventional values, and these values influence their role and functioning as parents (Kandel, 1990). For instance, substance using parents have displayed poor parenting skills, provided inadequate supervision of their children, and disciplined their children in a lax or coercive manner (Vaillant and Milofsky, 1982).

The relationships between alcohol use and relational quality are well documented. For instance, high levels of family dysfunction are related to alcohol use (McKay et al., 1992), and alcoholic couples have been characterized by interpersonal violence (Quigley and Leonard, 2000) and sexual dissatisfaction (O'Farrell et al., 1997). Spouses of alcoholics expressed greater dissatisfaction in all areas of family functioning than alcoholics (Suman and Nagalakshmi, 1995). This dissatisfaction may be reflected in the finding that both marital dissatisfaction and divorce rates are as much as seven times greater in alcoholics than the general population (Schafi et al., 1975). Medora and Woodward (1991) studied loneliness in alcoholics, finding significant negative relationships between the number of years alcohol was consumed and self-esteem, marital satisfaction, and loneliness. The relationship between alcohol use and relationship satisfaction may not be entirely linear. Under some circumstances, alcohol use has adaptive consequences (Steinglass, 1981) and has been associated with increased marital satisfaction. For example, Jacob et al. (1983) found that high alcohol consumption was associated with high levels of marital satisfaction in the spouses of steady drinkers, but not binge drinkers. An indirect effect or consequence of drug use may be difficulty in intimate relationship functioning among adult children of drug-using parents. Newcomb and Rickards (1995) found that parent drug-use problems predicted poor family support, and family support was strongly associated with good adult intimate relations for both men and women. Furthermore, for men, more parent drug-use problems reduced dyadic adjustment, increased dependence, and had a specific effect on reducing dating competence. For women, parent drug-use problems had no direct effects on adult intimacy or relationship variables.

4.4.2. Workplace

A large percentage of people in the workforce drink. Data from the National Household Survey on Drug Abuse (SAMHSA, 1998) indicated that almost 64% of full-time employed adults (26–34 years old) used alcohol in the past month. Those who use alcohol heavily are more likely to have increased absenteeism, and to have had at least three employers in the last year (SAMHSA, 1997). Several relationships have been found between alcohol use and employment. Those who endorse an escapist drinking style drink more alcohol in response to work stress (Grunberg et al., 1999). Moderate levels of consumption are associated with increased income, while heavy drinking may be detrimental to income levels (Mullahy and Sindelar, 1992). It is often hypothesized that alcoholics would have a less stable pattern of employment due to the adverse consequences of heavy drinking. In fact, failure to fulfill major role obligations (work, school, and home) is a criterion (DSM-IV) for alcohol abuse. The direct association between alcohol use and the hours/weeks worked, length of employment and/or job loss specifically due to drinking problems has not been widely studied (Mullahy and Sindelar, 1992). Low job satisfaction has been shown to be associated with alcoholism (Hingson et al., 1981). Galaif et al. (2001) found that polydrug problems were both predictors and consequences of work adjustment. Individuals abusing drugs were more likely to experience an erratic job pattern, less likely to adhere to societal norms, experience a less satisfying career, and have smaller support networks.

Overall, mixed results have been found regarding the association between drug use and work adjustment. Some investigations have documented inconsistent work histories, unemployment, work stress, absenteeism, tardiness, low quality work, job instability, work performance problems, and problems with job satisfaction among drug and alcohol users (Ames and James, 1987; Kandel, et al., 1986; Newcomb, 1988). Others have not found adverse effects on work adjustment (e.g., unemployment, job satisfaction, work performance) as a result of substance use (Bachman et al., 1984; Newcomb, 1988). Still, some researchers dispute the belief that drug use is a serious problem in the workplace (Newcomb, 1994b).

Tam et al. (2003) found that childhood adversity experiences were precursors to later alcohol and drug use in a sample of homeless adults. Subsequently, regular substance use was negatively associated with labor force participation and social service utilization.

5. CONCLUSIONS

Understanding and documenting both the short-term and long-term consequences of drug use and abuse are not as simple as it would appear. Drug use is intertwined with other norm-violating behaviors and attitudes (McGee and Newcomb, 1992) and it is difficult to disentangle consequences unique to drug use from aspects of general deviance (Newcomb, 1994). Further, drug use is only one influence that shapes and alters personal development. In fact, it is only one discrete component of the myriad biopsychosocial forces that forge a human being. Many of these may be far more potent and important than drug use in the evolving development and resulting outcome and qualities of a person and their life.

Disclaimer. This research was funded by grant DA 01070 from the National Institute on Drug Abuse.

REFERENCES

American Psychiatric Association (1994). *Diagnostic and Statistical Manual of Mental Disorders, Fourth Edition.* American Psychiatric Association, Washington, D.C.

Ames, G. M. and James, C. R. (1987). Heavy and problem drinking in an American blue collar population: Implications for prevention. *Social Science and Medicine* 25, pp. 949–960.

Apospori, E. A., Vega, W. A., Zimmerman, R. S., Warheit, G. J., and Gil, A. G. (1995). A longitudinal study of the conditional effects of deviant behavior on drug use among three racial/ethnic groups of adolescents. In: H. B. Kaplan (Ed.), *Drugs, Crime, and Other Deviant Adaptations: Longitudinal Studies* (pp. 211–230). Plenum, New York.

Bachman, J. G., O'Malley, P. M., and Johnston, L. D. (1984). Drug use among young adults: The impacts of role status and social environment. *Journal of Personality and Social Psychology* 47, pp. 629–645.

Baum-Baicker, C. (1985). The psychological benefits of moderate alcohol consumption: A review of the literature. *Drug and Alcohol Dependence* 15, pp. 305–322.

Baron, R. M., and Kenny, D. A. (1986). The moderator-mediator variable distinction in social psychological research: Conceptual, strategic, and statistical considerations. *Journal of Personality and Social Psychology* 51(60), pp. 1173–1182.

Brook, J. S., Brook, D. W., Rosen, Z., and Rabbitt, C. R. (2003). Earlier marijuana use and later problem behavior in Colombian youths. *Journal of the American Academy of Child and Adolescent Psychiatry* 42, pp. 485–492.

Brown A.S., Tapert S.F., Granholm E, and Delis D.C. (2000). Neurocognitive functioning of adolescents: effects of protracted alcohol use. *Alcohol Clinical and Experimental Research* 24, pp. 164–171.

Centers for Disease Control and Prevention (2003). HIV/AIDS among African Americans (online): http://www.cdc.gov/hiv/pubs/Facts/afam.htm.

Cherpitel, C. J. (2003). Changes in substance use associated with emergency room and primary care services utilization in the United States general population: 1995–2000. *American Journal of Drug and Alcohol Abuse* 29(4), pp. 789–802.

Christoffersen, M. N., Poulsen, H. D., and Nielsen, A. (2003). Attempted suicide among young people: Risk factors in a prospective register based study of Danish children born in 1966. *Acta Psychiatrica Scandinavica* 108(5), pp. 350–358.

Dackis, C. A. and Gold, M. S. (1983). Opiate addiction and depression–cause or effect? *Drug and Alcohol Dependence* 11, pp. 105–109.

Ellickson, P. L., Martino, S. C., and Collins, R. L. (2004). Marijuana use from adolescence to young adulthood: Multiple developmental trajectories and their associated outcomes. *Health Psychology* 23(3), pp. 299–307.

Galaif, E. R., Newcomb, M. D., and Vargas-Carmona, J. (2001). Prospective relationships between drug problems and work adjustment in a community sample of adults. *Journal of Applied Psychology* 86, pp. 337–350.

Grunberg, L., Moore, S., Anderson-Connolly, R., and Greenberg, E. (1999). Work stress and self-reported alcohol use: The moderating role of escapist reasons for drinking. *Journal of Occupational Health Psychology* 4(1), pp. 29–36.

Hanlon, T. E., Nurco, D. N., Kinlock, T. W., and Duszynski, K. R. (1990). Trends in criminal activity and drug use over an addiction career. *American Journal on Alcohol Abuse* 16, pp. 223–238.

Harrison, L. D. (1992). Trends in illicit drug use in the United States: Conflicting results from national surveys. *International Journal of the Addictions* 27, pp. 817–847.

Hingson, R. T. Mangione, T., and Barrett, J. (1981). Job characteristics and drinking practices in the Boston metropolitan area. *Journal of Studies on Alcohol* 42, pp. 725–738.

Holmbeck, G. (1997). Toward terminological, conceptual, and statistical clarity in the study of mediators and moderators: Examples from the child-clinical and pediatric psychology literatures. *Journal of Consulting and Clinical Psychology* 65(4), pp. 599–610.

Innes, C. A., and Greenfeld, L. A. (1990). *Violent State Prisoners And Their Victims (Special report).* U.S. Department of Justice, Washington, D.C.

Jacob, T., Dunn, N. J., and Leonard, K. (1983). Patterns of alcohol abuse and family stability. *Alcoholism: Clinical and Experimental Research* 7(4), pp. 382–385.

Kandel, D. B. (1990). Parenting styles, drug use, and children's adjustment in families of young adults. *Journal of Marriage and the Family* 52, pp. 183 196.

Kandel, D. B., Davies, M., Karus, D., and Yamaguchi, K. (1986). The consequences in young adulthood of adolescent drug involvement. *Archives of General Psychiatry* 43, pp. 746–754.

Kaplan, H. B. (1995). Drugs, crime, and other deviant adaptations. In: H. B. Kaplan (Ed.). *Drugs, Crime, and Other Deviant Adaptations: Longitudinal Studies* (pp. 3–46). Plenum, New York.

Kaplan, H. B., and Damphousse, K. R. (1995). Self-attitudes and antisocial personality as moderators of the drug use–violence relationship. In: H. B. Kaplan (Ed.), *Drugs, Crime, and Other Deviant Adaptations: Longitudinal Studies* (pp. 187–210). Plenum, New York.

Locke, T. F., and Newcomb, M. D. (2001). Alcohol problems and dysphoria: A longitudinal examination of gender differences from late adolescence to adulthood. *Psychology of Addictive Behaviors* 15(3), pp. 227–236.

Locke, T. F., and Newcomb, M. D. (2004). Childhood maltreatment, parent drug problems, polydrug problems, and parenting practices: A test of gender differences and four theoretical perspectives. *Journal of Family Psychology* 18(1), pp. 120–134.

Locke, T. F., Newcomb, M. D., and Goodyear, R. K. (in press). Childhood experiences and psychosocial influences on risky sexual behavior, condom use, and HIV attitudes/behaviors among Latino males. *Psychology of Men and Masculinity.*

Marlatt, G. A., Baer, J. S., Donovan, D. M., and Kivlahan, D. R. (1988). Addictive behaviors: Etiology and treatment. *Annual Review of Psychology* 19, pp. 223–252.

Mayes, L. C. (1995). Substance abuse and parenting. In: M. H. Bornstein (Ed.), *Handbook of Parenting, Vol. 4: Applied and Practical Parenting* (pp. 101–125). Erlbaum, Mahwah, NJ.

Medora, N. P., and Woodward, J. C. (1991). Factors associated with loneliness among alcoholics in rehabilitation centers. *Journal of Social Psychology* 131(6), pp. 769–779.

McGee, L., and Newcomb, M. D. (1992). General deviance syndrome: Expanded hierarchical evaluations at four ages from early adolescence to adulthood. *Journal of Consulting and Clinical Psychology* 60, pp. 766–776.

McKay, J. R., Longabaugh, R. Beattie, M. C. Maisto, S. A., and Noel, N. E. (1992). The relationship of pretreatment family functioning to drinking behavior during follow-up by alcoholic patients. *American Journal of Drug and Alcohol Abuse* 18(4), pp. 445–460.

Mokdad, A. H., Marks, J. S., Stroup, D. F., and Gerberding, J. L. (2004). Actual causes of death in the United States, 2000. *Journal of the American Medical Association* 291(10), pp. 1238–1245.

Mullahy, J., and Sindelar, J. (1992). Effects of alcohol on labor market success: Income, earnings, labor supply and occupation. *Alcohol Health and Research World* 16(2):134–139.

The National Institute on Drug Abuse (NIDA) (2003, June). NIDA InfoFacts. http://www.drugabuse. gov/Infofax/DrugAbuse.html.

The National Institute on Alcohol Abuse and Alcoholism (NIAAA) (2004). NIAAA Quick Facts http:// www.niaaa.nih.gov/databases/qf.htm.

Newcomb, M. D. (1988). *Drug Use in the Workplace: Risk Factors for Disruptive Substance Use Among Young Adults.* Auburn House, Dover, MA.

Newcomb, M. D. (1994). Drug use and intimate relationships among women and men: Separating specific from general effects in prospective data using structural equations models. *Journal of Consulting and Clinical Psychology* 62, pp. 463–476.

Newcomb, M. D. (1994b). Prevalence of drug use in the workplace: Cause for concern or irrational hysteria? *Journal of Drug Issues* 24, pp. 403–416.

Newcomb, M. D. (1997). Psychosocial predictors and consequences of drug use: A developmental perspective within a prospective study. *Journal of Addictive Diseases* 16, pp. 51–89.

Newcomb M. D. (2004). *Understanding Drug Use as a Developmental and Mediating Process: Theoretical Considerations and Empirical Examples.* Paper presented at Beyond the Drug: APSAD 2004 National Conference. Perth, Australia.

Newcomb, M. D., Abbott, R. D., Catalano, R. F., Hawkins, J. D., Battin-Pearson, S. R., and Hill, K. (2002). Mediational and deviance theories of late high school failure: Process roles of structural strains, academic competence, and general versus specific problem behaviors. *Journal of Counseling Psychology* 49, pp. 172–186.

Newcomb, M. D., and Bentler, P. M. (1987). The impact of late adolescent substance use on young adult health status and utilization of health services: A structural equation model over four years. *Social Science and Medicine* 24, pp. 71–82.

Newcomb, M. D., and Bentler, P. M. (1988). *Consequences of Adolescent Drug Use: Impact on the Lives of Young Adults.* Sage Publications, Beverly Hills, CA.

Newcomb, M. D., Bentler, P. M. and Collins, C. (1986). Alcohol use and dissatisfaction with self and life: A longitudinal analysis of young adults. *Journal of Drug Issues* 16, pp. 479–494.

Newcomb, M. D., and Jack, L. E. (1995). Drug use, agency, and communality: Causes and consequences among adults. *Psychology of Addictive Behaviors*, pp. 967–982.

Newcomb, M. D., and Galaif, E. R., and Vargas-Carmona, J. (2001). The drug-crime nexus among a community sample of adults. *Psychology of Addictive Behaviors* 15, pp. 185–193.

Newcomb, M. D., and Locke, T. F., and Good year, R. K. (2003). Childhood experiences and psychosocial influences on HIV risk among adolescent Latinas in Southern California. *Cultural Diversity and Ethnic Minority Psychology* 9, pp. 219–235.

Newcomb, M. D., and Loeb, T. B. (1999). Poor parenting as an adult problem behavior: General deviance, deviant attitudes, inadequate family support/bonding, or just bad parents? *Journal of Family Psychology* 13, pp. 175–193.

Newcomb, M. D., and Rickards, S. (1995). Parent drug-use problems and adult intimate relations: Associations among community samples of young adult women and men. *Journal of Counseling Psychology* 42(2), pp. 141–154.

Newcomb, M. D., Scheier, L. M., and Bentler, P. M. (1993). Effects of adolescent drug use on adult mental health: A prospective study of a community sample. *Experimental and Clinical Psychopharmacology* 1, pp. 215–241.

Newcomb, M. D., Vargas-Carmona, J. and Galaif, E. R. (1999). Drug problems and psychological distress among a community sample of adults: Predictors, consequences, or confound? *Journal of Community Psychology* 27, pp. 405–429.

O'Farrell, T. J., Choquette, K. A., Cutter, H., G., and Birchler, G. R. (1997). Sexual satisfaction and dysfunction in marriages of male alcoholics: Comparison with nonalcoholic martially conflicted and nonconflicted couples. *Journal of Studies on Alcohol* 58(1), pp. 91–99.

Palepu, A., Horton, N. J., Tibbetts, N., Dukes, K., Meli, S., and Samet, J.H. (2003). Substance abuse treatment and emergency department utilization among a cohort of HIV-infected persons with alcohol problems. *Journal of Substance Abuse Treatment* 25(1), pp. 37–42.

Pencer, A. and Addington, J. (2003). Substance use and cognition in early psychosis. *Journal of Psychiatry and Neuroscience* 28(1), pp. 48–54.

Quigley, B. M., and Leonard, K. E. (2000). Alcohol and the continuation of early marital aggression. *Alcoholism: Clinical and Experimental Research* 24(7), pp. 1003–1010.

Saunders, D. R. (1956). Moderator variables in prediction. *Educational and Psychological Measurement* 16, pp. 209–222.

SAMHSA [Substance Abuse and Mental Health Service Administration] (1997). *Worker Drug Use and Workplace Policies and Programs: Results from the 1994 and 1997 National Household Survey on Drug Abuse*. US Government Printing Office, Washington, D.C.

SAMHSA [Substance Abuse and Mental Health Service Administration] (1998). *National Household Survey on Drug Abuse: Main Findings 1992*. US Government Printing Office, Washington, D.C.

Schafi, M., Lavely, R., and Jaffe, R. (1975). Medication and the prevention of alcohol abuse. *American Journal of Psychiatry* 132(9), pp. 942–945.

Schuckit, M. A. (1986). Genetic and clinical implications of alcoholism and affective disorder. *American Journal of Psychiatry* 143(2), pp. 140–147.

Shedler, J and Block, J. (1990). Adolescent drug use and psychological health: A longitudinal inquiry. *American Psychologist* 45(5), pp. 612–630.

Stein, J. A., Newcomb, M. D., and Bentler, P. M. (1988). Structure of drug use behaviors and consequences among young adults: A multitrait-multimethod assessment of frequency, quantity, worksite, and problematic substance use. *Journal of Applied Psychology* 73, pp. 595–605.

Steinglass, P. (1981). The alcoholic family at home: Patterns of interaction in dry, wet, and transitional stages of alcoholism. *Archives of General Psychiatry* 38(5) pp. 578–584.

Suman, L. N., and Nagalakshmi, S. V. (1995). Family interaction patterns in alcoholic families. *NIMHANS Journal* 13(1), pp. 47–52.

Tam, T. W., Zlotnick, C., and Robertson, M. J. (2003). Longitudinal perspective: Adverse childhood events, substance use, and labor force participation among homeless adults. *American Journal of Drug and Alcohol Abuse* 29(4), pp. 829–846.

Tapert, S. F., Aarons, G. A., Sedlar, G. R., and Brown, S. A. (2001). Adolescent substance abuse and sexual risk-taking behavior. *Journal of Adolescent Health* 28(3), pp. 181–189.

Testa, M. and Collins, R. L. (1997). Alcohol and risky sexual behavior: Event-based analyses among a sample of high-risk women. *Psychology of Addictive Behaviors* 11(3), pp. 190–201.

Vaillant, G. E. (1993). Is alcoholism more often the cause or the result of depression? *Harvard Review of Psychiatry* 1(2), pp. 94–99.

Vaillant, G. E. (1995). *The Natural History of Alcoholism Revisited*. Harvard University Press, Cambridge, MA.

Vaillant, G.E. and Milofsky, E.S. (1982). The etiology of alcoholism: A prospective viewpoint. *American Psychologist* 37, pp. 494–503.

White, A. M. (2004) http://www.duke.edu/~amwhite/index.html.

Zedeck, S. (1971). Problems with the use of "moderator" variables. *Psychological Bulletin* 76, pp. 295–310.

B

Epidemiological Methods

5

Use of Archival Data

Zili Sloboda, Rebecca McKetin and Nicholas J. Kozel

ZILI SLOBODA • Institute for Health and Social Policy, The University of Akron
REBECCA McKETIN • National Drug and Alcohol Research Centre, University of New South
Wales Sydney
NICHOLAS J. KOZEL • Consultant, Bangkok, Thailand; formerly Associate Director, Division of
Epidemiology and Prevention Research, National Institute on Drug Abuse

1. INTRODUCTION

The foregoing section laid out the natural history of drug use and abuse including a discussion of the origins and pathways and the associated health, social, and psychological consequences. This section will address the methods most often used by drug abuse epidemiologists to both describe the problem within a defined geographic area or population and to understand the nature of the problem. The first chapter in this section discusses the most basic epidemiologic approach used to define the parameters of a drug problem, the use of archival or existing data. In this chapter, the need for multiple sources of information on drug use is recommended in response to the stigmatized nature of drug abuse in most societies which often limits identification through self-report as individuals seek to avoid incriminating themselves. Even where laws against the possession, sales or use of drugs of abuse are not fully enforced, there is usually social stigma against drug users, thus inhibiting acknowledgement of such use.

Accessing vulnerable or susceptible persons or persons who are actually affected with a health problem is a difficult challenge for all epidemiologists and not limited to those addressing drug abuse. Researchers interested in mental health problems, cancer, heart disease, and most other medical problems face similar barriers. For some of these conditions, registries, reports or insurance billing information represent the primary source of information on affected cases. An excellent example of this approach is the use of Surveillance, Epidemiology, and End Result (SEER) data for cancer incidence and mortality (National Cancer Institute). Currently SEER receives reports of cases from 14 population-based areas including States, counties, and extended metropolitan regions. Information from SEER is projected for all of the United States. Another example of this approach is for HIV infection and AIDS. The Centers for Disease Prevention and Control have established registries within State-level health departments that receive reports of infected persons (Centers for Disease Control and Prevention, 2001). Both the SEER and HIV registries begin with reports that have minimal information and add subsequent information from medical records or investigative summaries (Gornick et al., 2004). For other medical problems, surveys are used to determine the extent of these problems in general populations, usually asking the respondents if they have the problem or if they have symptoms that may or may not be both sensitive and specific to the index problem. These types of studies may follow a series of cohorts recruited from a general population living in defined areas every year or less frequently. A good example is the renowned Framingham study in which study participants are being followed every two years with questionnaires and medical examinations (National Heart, Lung, and Blood Institute). The first cohort established in 1948 consisted of over 5,000 residents between the ages of 30 and 62. The second consisted of the children of the first cohort, established in 1971. Currently, the researchers are recruiting the children of the second cohort.

Data from the study have contributed greatly to our knowledge about the risks for heart disease (e.g., Lloyd-Jones et al., 2004). Other researchers have studied cohorts of persons who have been identified as being at risk for disease by virtue of their family history or life styles. These longitudinal studies determine the specific factors that precipitate or protect from disease manifestation, morbidity, and mortality.

This chapter will focus on the use of archival data in epidemiologic systems to monitor and understand the drug abuse situation. The first section will describe potential sources of archival data and discuss their advantages and disadvantages. The second section will present an example of a successful surveillance system, the Community Epidemiology Work Group (CEWG) and the contributions this system has made to our understanding of drug abuse in the United States. Finally, the chapter will conclude with suggestions as to how archival data can be used for policy.

2.   SOURCES OF ARCHIVAL DATA

Archival data consist of information maintained by agencies that provide services to drug abusers, such as drug abuse treatment programs, hospital emergency rooms and clinics, medical examiners or coroner's offices, social service organizations as well as law enforcement and criminal justice agencies. Through the review of archival data it is possible to determine: (1) the nature of the drug use problem, i.e., types of drugs being used, methods of use, and frequency of use and (2) the characteristics of those who use drugs. The use of such data has many advantages. Archival data are both inexpensive and generally easy to access. However, there are inherent biases associated with archival data as the information included on routine records or statistical reports may be limited or unverified. For example, emergency room personnel do not routinely ask about or test for drugs that may be used by the patients they serve and unless the episode is related to a drug-related problem, may fail to even consider the involvement of drugs. Yet archival data are rich sources of information particularly for communities and countries that do not have the resources for other epidemiologic studies. In addition, if archival data are standardized and routine, they can serve as a significant part of a more comprehensive surveillance system and over time have the potential for identifying emergent new drug use patterns, including new drugs of abuse, new methods for using existing drugs, and new populations involved in the use of drugs. Both the World Health Organization and the United Nations suggest that archival data should be one component of a multiple component epidemiologic information system (WHO, 2000; United Nations, 2003) that includes both household and school surveys and studies of special populations. To be effective these data sources should form an integrated information system of experts that collects and reviews the data on a regular basis.

Each geographic or political community varies in the types of data that would be readily available as input into any drug use information system. Generally, the sources of these data are obvious, but some are less so. Most guides or manuals, such as the WHO Guide to Drug Abuse Epidemiology (World Health Organization, 2000) and the UN's Global Assessment Program's Toolkit, Module 1 (United Nations, 2003), suggest ways to make an inventory of these resources. How and whether drug use patterns will be reflected in archival data depends on the natural history of local drug use patterns, the types of services available to drug users, and the type of information collected through existing data collection systems. For this reason it is important to gain an understanding of the local drug situation and how this might be captured through archival data sources. Methods to do this include a review of any available data on the natural history of drug use, talking with local providers of services to drug users, and holding focus groups with drug users. One caution in the selection of these "informants" is that the lifestyles of different types of drug users may vary widely due to the physiological effects of the drugs used, the costs and availability of the drugs, and numerous other social, psychological, physical and environmental factors.

The circumstances that prompt drug users into a treatment service situation may not be universal. The literature does indicate that not all drug users come into contact with service agencies and many manage their drug use without any apparent need for treatment or medical assistance and without coming to the attention of law enforcement. As Hser et al. indicate in their chapter in this publication, most natural history studies begin with groups of drug users already identified through treatment or the criminal justice system. They also state that it is likely that the more severe or problematic drug users will have contact with social service, health, or criminal justice agencies. There is a dearth of information in the literature regarding drug users' utilization and contact with any of these agencies. Nurco and his colleagues (1984, 1988) have studied the addiction careers of different groups of narcotic users and provide findings on the association between periods of addiction and involvement in crime. They find that criminal activities decrease during periods of nonaddiction. Other studies have found that drug users differ in their use of medical services. Those with more severe problems, including psychosocial issues, are more likely to use emergency and inpatient services than other groups of drug users or neighborhood control non-drug users (French et al., 2000; Reynolds et al., 2003). Furthermore, as with the general population, those with more resources will have access to more services. Finally, there are differences in service utilization by gender and ethnicity (Brown et al., 1993). All these factors must be considered when accessing archival data to correct the bias or, at least, to be cognizant that biases are present.

There are six primary sources of archival data that are generally included in most information systems on drug use. They each have their advantages and disadvantages. These are: (1) drug treatment programs, (2) hospital admissions and emergency rooms/departments logs, (3) public health or infectious disease registries, (4) poison control centers, (5) medical examiners/coroners offices, and (6) criminal justice/law enforcement agencies. These are good sources of information, but each also has certain limitations that are discussed below. Probably the greatest limitations to these sources are: (1) they include persons who may have used drugs only once, (2) they are not "population-based", i.e. prevalence and incidence rates of drug use for the general population can not be calculated directly from these numbers, (3) a drug user could appear multiple times in multiple records, since they are not independent of each other, and (4) they are sensitive to administrative and policy changes, e.g. if a city official in response to public opinion orders a crack-down on drug users, the numbers of arrests may increase representing a change in implementation of law and not necessarily an increase in drug use.

2.1. Drug Treatment Programs

The availability of treatment for drug use varies across communities and includes a range of possibilities from public, free-standing programs to private regimens within existing general or specialty clinic practice (Substance Abuse and Mental Health Services Administration, 2003). Therefore, it is important when considering drug use treatment resources to develop a list of facilities where drug users would go for treatment. In most communities where no treatment programs are readily available, nearby general, mental health, or psychiatric hospitals may provide treatment services to local residents. Treatment data collection systems usually have a pragmatic focus on collecting data from a defined set of treatment services rather than being all inclusive

The major advantage of accessing drug treatment facilities is that they are more likely than other types of facilities to collect useful information on drug use patterns, since their focus is drug abuse. In addition to having information on the demographic characteristics of their patients including their place of residence, they should have detailed data on the types of drugs being used, the frequency of their use, the mode of drug administration, and about associated social, economic, psychological, and health problems, since this information is needed for deciding on treatment strategies.

Unfortunately, there are a number of potential disadvantages associated with treatment data. For instance, the treatment provider may be interested solely in the patients' drug of choice or the patients' self-determined primary drug problem and may not ask about the use of other types of drugs or about the patients' histories with drugs and other substances, such as alcohol and tobacco. Patients involved in public programs may have different drug using patterns, problems, and histories from those attending private programs/regimens. Also, those in treatment may not be representative of drug users in general. For instance, Price et al. (2001) found that at the time of their 1997 follow-up survey of a cohort of drug abusers recruited in the early 1970s, fewer than 9 percent of those admitting to drug use were in any type of treatment program. In addition, those in treatment may also be older and their drug use may not represent emergent patterns of use. Often data on drug treatment distinguishes between new treatment clients and repeat admissions to help discern recent drug trends, although there typically remains a lag between onset of an emergent drug practice and entry into treatment. Finally, not all of those presenting for treatment are self-referred or self-motivated. A sufficient portion of these admissions may be in treatment as an alternative to jail and possibly may not be as involved with drugs as the general drug using population (Friedmann et al., 2003; Joe et al., 1999). For these reasons, it is important to have a good understanding as to how people come to treatment and how information regarding drug use is recorded. Interpretation of treatment data should also consider shifts in drug treatment provision, such as implementation of a new treatment modality or improved access to treatment that may increase the number of people entering drug treatment. Large scale shifts in treatment provision may occur in response to growing or changing drug trends, and it can difficult to tease out the relative contribution of drug use trends per se over that of shifts in service provision.

2.2.   Hospital Admissions and Emergency Department Logs

The process of maintaining records in hospitals varies across countries. In the United States, hospital admissions and discharges are reported centrally and the International Classification of Diseases is used to code the diagnosis associated with each hospital stay. Emergency or urgent care episodes generally include cases of accidents, suicides, homicides as well as those situations when someone is ill and has no ready access to medical care. As discussed above, this would be the situation for most problematic drug users.

Among the advantages of using hospital and emergency department information is that it is here that new drugs of abuse and new ways of using drugs may be observed as naïve drug users may have negative physical reactions to these new drugs, requiring medical attention. In addition, drug users who may not come to the attention of the criminal justice system or admit themselves to treatment may use the emergency department for their health care. The major disadvantage of using hospital and emergency department records is unless drug use in obvious, i.e. drug use is the primary, secondary or tertiary reason for the visit, staff may not ask about it. In addition, some drugs may not cause the kind of consequences which require emergency treatment, even though they may be of great concern to the community. A case in point is ecstasy. In the absence of laboratory tests of body fluids, drugs also may go undetected and, thus, unreported because the patient or whoever provided the initial information was unaware that the drug ingested was contaminated with other substances. This type of situation occurred relatively frequently in the past when marijuana was reported as the cause for emergency room presentation when, in fact, the marijuana had been contaminated with phencyclidine (PCP) which was a more likely candidate for causing the primary condition requiring emergency attention. Thus, similar to treatment data, the service delivery process at the care giving facility needs to be understood fully in order to avoid drawing inaccurate conclusions from the records.

2.3. Public Health Reports of Infectious Diseases

Reporting the diagnosis of certain infectious diseases is required in many communities and in many countries. Generally, reportable infectious diseases are found at high rates among drug abusers including human immunodeficiency virus (HIV) infection or acquired immunodeficiency syndrome (AIDS), hepatitis A, B, C, and Delta; tuberculosis, and sexually transmitted diseases. Usually inquiries are made as to the mode of transmission and as tracing and notification are essential components of these programs, demographic information should be available for each case.

As in the case of hospital and emergency department information, these reporting systems will include drug users who may not appear in any other service agency records. In addition, monitoring these systems on a routine basis will detect increases of the spread of infection and identify those populations or areas to target interventions. However, these systems may not request information on drug use or, if they do ask about drug using behaviors, they may not provide much detail (Klevens et al., 2001).

2.4. Poison Control Reports

Both medical personnel and the public report negative health effects of drugs and other substances to poison control centers. The broad based reporting provides valuable information on both emergent and existing drug use practices. An example of an emergent problem discovered through reports from a poison control center was noted at a December 1998 meeting of the Community Epidemiology Work Group in Miami in which the use of gamma-hydroxybutyrate (GHB) and its precursor gamma-butyrolactone (GBL) were reported being used in combination with 3, 4-methylenedioxymethamphetamine, also known as MDMA, X, and ecstasy, in clubs and at dance parties, such as raves (National Institute on Drug Abuse, 1999). The report also stated that GHB was implicated in both the onset of serious illness and death. The major limitation of these reporting systems is that the reports are of single drug use episodes, do not necessarily reflect long-term drug use or widespread drug use patterns, and may lack detailed information regarding the specifics of drug use to understand what populations are represented in the reports.

2.5.   Medical Examiners/Coroners Reports

In most locales, medical examiners and coroners are responsible for investigating sudden and unexpected as well as violent deaths. As legal issues are at stake, they are responsible for compiling sufficient evidence to support their determination of cause of death. In many countries, their reports of cause of death are an important part of the nation's vital statistics. However, there is great variation across communities, and even within communities, in the training of medical examiners/coroners and in their level of expertise and interest in issues, such as drug use. Medical examiners/coroners in different jurisdictions may use different criteria for defining drug-related deaths and have different levels of experience in recognizing these deaths. For these reasons, the quality of reports of cause of death may not be uniform across jurisdictions (Shai, 1994; Smith Sehden and Hutchins, 2001). In addition, not all deaths are thoroughly investigated and even, in cases where all deaths are investigated, toxicology screens to determine the use of drugs are not always ordered. Therefore, it is important to know the processes used by the medical examiner's office when accessing death reports. Most drug use data systems include information on the direct and indirect causes of death, but unless the information on drug use is collected, information for deaths among drug users due to natural causes or other diseases may not be included. Drug users may die from a number of reasons related directly to drug use as in the case of drug poisoning or overdose. Or the cause of death may be indirectly linked to drug use, such as homicide, suicide, and AIDS or other infection, e.g., sepsis, bacterial endocarditis. Therefore it is important to distinguish between deaths caused by drugs (e.g., overdose or poisoning by drugs) and those deaths where drug use was an in-direct cause. There are clear advantages to this source of information on drug use practices, similar to those of the other medical/health sources mentioned above. However, the reporting system will be substantially affected due to the lack of medical training in some offices, the failure to conduct posthumous investigations, lack of drug testing and, in addition, the limitations imposed by rules concerning which deaths are referred to the medical examiner/coroner for autopsy. Drug-related deaths data are also more reflective of drugs or combinations of drugs that are associated with higher risk of mortality. It is also important to recognize that most death data only indicate one drug as the primary cause of death, while toxicology results often indicate the presence of several drugs that may have cumulatively resulted in death.

2.6.   Law Enforcement

The illegal nature of drug use in most countries will also place drug users at risk of arrest. Law enforcement agencies not only can provide information about people arrested for drug use or non-drug use crimes, but also they often seize drugs and in some cases, analyze the seized drugs to determine the type of drug and purity levels. Law enforcement agencies may also keep track of the street prices of drugs and have a better understanding as to how drugs are marketed. Information from law enforcement agencies has the advantage that it may capture a different segment of the drug using population to that captured through treatment services or other general health services; however, arrest data tend to over-represent males and obviously those who are criminally involved. One major disadvantage of arrest data is bias by the imposition of policing operations that target particular types of drugs or drug markets and strategic directions taken in response to public outcry or a political need to respond to a particular drug problem. Purity and price data can also be influenced by the focus of the policing activity while it is also important to consider sampling issues with price and purity data. Price data from law enforcement may be based on a small number of reports and may not be indicative of street level prices. Similarly not all drug seizures may be analyzed for purity: this may be related to local legislations around the necessity to verify purity and constituents of drugs seized. Lack of confirmation of drug seizure content can also affect the way drug trends are reflected in arrest statistics. Finally, as in many cases drug use carries great social stigma, those arrestees from the higher socioeconomic groups may be able to have their arrest records expunged or have the reason for arrest altered. Despite these weaknesses, law enforcement data provide an important adjunct to other data sources by capturing drug users who may not be represented in health data sources and also in understanding factors about the drug market that may influence consumption patterns.

2.7. Overcoming Limitations of Existing Data

Experience with existing drug abuse data and information systems has lead to a variety of methods being implemented to address their limitations. In general, there are two approaches used to collect the information needed to assess the drug use situation in a community. One is to collect information after the fact, either selecting time periods over the calendar year or selecting a random or systematic sample of records, such as hospital discharges, emergency logs, or arrests and to have trained staff abstract these records. The second approach is to be more proactive in collecting the information by interviewing persons admitted or discharged from a hospital, contacting the emergency department staff, or being present at the time of processing an arrest. This approach requires having trained staff available 24 hours a day or using some other time schedule to interview patients or arrestees, using the universe or a sample of the population, about their drug use and reasons for making their agency contact. There are significant costs associated with the two approaches both in terms of training and manpower. When using either, it is important to account for variations in contacts, such as seasons or holidays and that the periods of data collection are sufficient to detect drug use. In addition, a denominator of all contacts, both drug users and non-users should be obtained as a basis for computation of population rates.

If agency reports are being used, it is important to work with the responsible agency staff to understand how the information is collected and inquiries should be made concerning whether reporting forms could be revised to include more detailed information about drug use, such as the type of drugs used, mode of ingestion (e.g., injecting, snorting, smoking, swallowing), frequency of use, and longevity of use. Understandably, most agencies would be resistant to making changes. For this reason, having agency representatives form a community-based data group that reviews the information from multiple sources may serve to stimulate change. The development of an information group or network allows access to a wide-range of data sources and any interpretation of data output represents the viewpoints of a number of community sectors. Thus, it is recommended that when forming these groups participating members are recruited from a variety of diverse agencies. The major objectives of these networks should include defining the characteristics of the drug use problem in the community and detecting emergent drug patterns in order to monitor them and to prevent their spread. In order to achieve these aims, it is important to collect data over sequential time periods, e.g. quarterly, semi-annually, or annually, and to interpret any observed changes to consider if they truly represent alterations of drug use patterns or if they are the artifact of administrative decisions about agency operations. If the observed change is consistent across all reporting sources, there will be more confidence in accepting the change as real.

3. THE COMMUNITY EPIDEMIOLOGY WORK GROUP: AN EXAMPLE

One of the authors (Kozel) of this chapter is considered the founder of the Community Epidemiology Work Group (CEWG) that is supported by the National Institute on Drug Abuse (NIDA). The CEWG was established in 1976 as a group of epidemiology experts representing cities across the United States. Twenty-one city representatives participate in the group at the time of the writing of this chapter many of whom have been involved with the group for ten years or more. The group meets twice a year, in June and December, when each member presents a report of information from several sources. Several articles have been published about the CEWG, describing its operation and its findings (Kozel, 1993; Sloboda and Kozel, 2003). The CEWG members generally use existing reports from local agencies within their cities. The challenge to the CEWG has been to summarize this information with its varying definitions of terms and emphases. In an attempt to standardize reporting procedures, for more than 25 years the membership of the CEWG along with the NIDA staff have developed routine reporting formats, so that an equivalent, minimal data set is collected. To enrich this basic information, the members draw on the findings of ongoing research or of periodic school or household surveys, and often adding ethnographic or focus group information that provides context to the primarily quantitatively-based drug abuse "picture" in their areas.

At each meeting, after the members briefly discuss the current status and trends of drug use, the group will seek commonalities or discuss differences particularly of any change in drug use practices, such as the introduction of a new drug, a new way of using an existing drug, or new population groups using a drug. The members also discuss gaps in their data, set priorities as to which gaps need to be addressed, and develop ways as to how this can be done. Oftentimes one or more members will introduce and suggest a new resource to the others while sharing what additional or confirmatory information this source provides.

The CEWG model can be applied at different geopolitical levels from local communities, to countries, or to a region. Country or regional work groups would include representatives of smaller systems or networks and each representative would present the findings from his or her network. The aims of these larger groups are to seek unique and common trends across a large geographic area and to understand the factors influencing differences when they occur.

Although the CEWG is U.S.-based, over the years an international component has been added so that epidemiologists, researchers, and policy makers from other countries have an opportunity to report on drug use trends in their communities or countries. Exposure to the operation of the CEWG has led to a number of countries adopting the approach. For instance, the Ministerial Conference of the Pompidou Group created an Epidemiology Expert Group in 1982 to develop monitoring systems to evaluate the drug abuse and related problems in Europe. Other countries that have established similar groups include Mexico, Canada, and South Africa. Regional groups include the Americas and the Caribbean under the sponsorship of the Organization of American States, South and Southeast Asia under the sponsorship of the United Nations Office on Drugs and Crime—Regional Centre for East Asia and the Pacific, and the Southern African Development Community countries under the sponsorship of the European Communities. In addition, the Headquarters of the United Nations Office on Drugs and Crime (2003) has developed a manual for self-training in methods for establishing and implementing similar data systems.

The potential of an information system such as the CEWG addresses at least four aspects: (1) defining emergent drug use trends, (2) examining the time-space relationship of drug use patterns, (3) generating research questions, and (4) contributing to epidemiologic methods.

3.1. Emergent Trends

New trends in drug use patterns generally are observed first by law enforcement and emergency department staff. Sloboda and Kozel (2003) suggest that these new trends occur among existing drug using populations and that it may take one to two years before they are observed within a general population. As stated above emergent patterns of drug use may include new types or formulations of drugs, new methods for using existing drugs, new population groups using existing drugs, or some combination of all three possibilities. Examples of new drugs detected through the CEWG have been reported for methaqualone (Quaalude) in the 1970s, crack-cocaine in the 1980s, Rohypnol in the 1990s, and GHB and OxyContin in the late 1990s and early 2000s. At first these new drugs were observed in one or more cities. Once mentioned at the CEWG meeting, members went back to their colleagues and data sources to determine if these drugs were showing up in their areas. Over time, the members were able to document the spread of the use of these drugs and the health problems associated with their use. With this information it was possible to involve public health agencies to alert hospitals and law enforcement agencies and through print and electronic media to educate the public about these drugs and the consequences of their use.

Not only have new types of drugs been detected by CEWG members but also they have documented new ways to administer drugs. The use of blunts, i.e., marijuana-filled cigars, was noted in the early 1990s among African-American youth in cities in the northeast region of the country before spreading to other cities. Blunts combined with alcohol, which became culturally embedded as a 40 ounce can of malt liquor, became so prevalent that the pattern was included in movies and rap music. Other examples of new administration practices include snorting of heroin as a purer version of the drug was made available from Colombia and injecting crack cocaine when users discovered they could dissolve the drug in lemon juice or vinegar (Sloboda and Kozel, 2003).

Lastly, new subpopulations involved with specific drug use practices have been observed at the CEWG meetings. Several examples have been presented in Sloboda and Kozel (2003). Among these is the movement of heroin from urban to suburban areas as snorting the purer form became more acceptable in the 1990s. Another example has been the spread of methamphetamine use from more geographically defined areas around cities in the west and southwest and in rural areas to almost every part of the country and moving from outlaw motorcycle gangs and certain Asian groups to more diverse populations, including young people. It was possible to attribute these changes when information from the Drug Enforcement Administration was reviewed showing that the source of the new waves of methamphetamines came from Mexico and was distributed along marijuana trafficking routes.

3.2.   Time-Space Relationship of Drug Use Patterns

As with other public health issues, there is an apparent time-space relationship to various forms of drug use. There is a commonality in the use of drugs, such as marijuana, cocaine, and heroin across and within countries, the popularity of these drugs may rise and fall depending on their availability, purity, price, and on public perceptions regarding their social acceptability and the associated serious nature of the consequences of their use. Yet, some drugs are notably endemic to a particular geographic area or may be popular at certain periods of time. Examples of endemic drugs are "ice" in Hawaii and PCP in Washington, D.C. While many large cities were dealing with an epidemic of crack-cocaine, it did not make an appearance in Chicago until several years later. Certainly environmental factors, particularly drug markets and trafficking, explain much of the time-space relationship that has been observed consistently by the CEWG members. What is not as clear is what forces work to move new drugs and administration styles across boundaries and to more diverse populations. Clearly the expansion of interstate highways and movement of goods and people and the internet and media suggest an explanation to the "how" question, but the "why" of adopting these new patterns is not so apparent and warrants further investigation.

3.3.   Generating Research Questions

The above discussions regarding emergent new problems and their spread raise important questions. Some of these have been addressed first through ethnographic or qualitative studies and focus groups. This exploratory work helped refine research questions and suggest population and sampling plans that were incorporated into further research. An excellent example of such an approach surrounded the issue of the spread of methamphetamines that is described more fully by Pach and Gorman (2003). A group of ethnographers conducted a study using a standard approach in six cities. The cities were selected on the basis of how extensive the problem was—endemic, emergent, or unclear. This research provided insights into the new populations affected by methamphetamines and into the specific consequences of their use. Several other areas of research raised by the information presented by the CEWG are discussed in Sloboda and Kozel (2003).

3.4.   Contributions of the CEWG to Drug Abuse Epidemiologic Methods

Several epidemiologic methods have evolved through the processes of the CEWG. The most dominant has been the ability to develop a sound description of the drug abuse situation within a geographic area. The systematic integration of data from a variety of sources into reporting formats that can be reviewed and discussed have empowered communities to document drug abuse problems and to provide planners and policy makers with information that helps to define prevention and treatment needs. In addition, the CEWG has shown how existing data sets can be used across time and geography to document emergent problems. Finally, through the research that has been generated by the CEWG, an integrated quantitative and qualitative approach has been developed that has been embraced by drug abuse epidemiologists (Agar and Kozel, 1999; Sterk and Elifson, Chapter 9, herein).

4. CONCLUSIONS

Drug abuse has become recognized as a public health problem around the globe by both the United Nations and the World Health Organization. But even in the most accepting of countries the nature of drug abuse poses a barrier to the use of traditional public health epidemiologic approaches. Part of that nature is how it can and has changed over time, presenting public health workers with new drugs of abuse, new and sometimes very dangerous methods for drug administration, and involving more vulnerable populations. At times these changes are contained and short-lived, but many times they spread across population groups and become endemic over years. The Community Epidemiology Work Group has become an important tool to be used with others from the more traditional epidemiologic armatarium to assess drug abuse at the local, regional, national, and international levels. The information gathered describes current drug use patterns and can suggest potential future issues. It can also generate questions or issues that can be further researched. Finally, it serves as a resource for public health planners and policy makers to plan for services and the allocation of resources. Clearly, the rapid diffusion of the CEWG model to other countries and regions of the world support the efficacy of this approach.

REFERENCES

Agar, M.H. and Kozel, N.J. (1999). Ethnography and substance use: talking numbers. Introduction. Substance Use and Misuse 34(14), pp. 1935–1949.

Bless, R. (2003). Experiences of the pompidou group multi-city network 1983–2002. *Bulletin on Narcotics* LV(1 and 2), pp. 31–40.

Brown, L.S., Jr., Alterman, A.I., Rutherford, M.J., Cacciola, J.S., and Zaballero, A.R. (1993). Addiction Severity Index Scores of Four Racial/Ethnic and Gender Groups of Methadone Maintenance Patients. *Journal of Substance Abuse* 5(3), pp. 269–279.

Centers for Disease Control and Prevention (2001). *AIDS Public Information Data Set–December 2001*. Atlanta, Georgia.

French, M.T., McGeary, K.A., Chitwood, D.D., and McCoy, C.B. (2000). Chronic illicit drug use, health services utilization and the cost of medical care. *Social Science and Medicine* 50(12), pp. 1703–1713.

Friedmann, P.D., Lemon, S.C., Stein, M.D. and D'Aunno, T.A. (2003). Community referral sources and entry of treatment-naive clients into outpatient addiction treatment. *American Journal of Drug and Alcohol Abuse* 29(1), pp. 105–115.

Gornick, M.E., Eggers, P.W., and Riley, G.F. (2004). Associations of race, education, and patterns of preventive service use with stage of cancer at time of diagnosis. *Health Services Research* 39(5), 1403–1428.

Hser, Y-I., Longshore, D., and Anglin, M.D. (2005). Studying the natural history of drug use. In: Sloboda, Z. (Ed.) *Epidemiology of Drug Abuse*. Kluwer Academic/Plenum Publishers, New York.

Joe, G.W., Simpson, D.D., and Broome, K.M. (1999). Retention and patient engagement models for different treatment modalities in DATOS. *Drug and Alcohol Dependence* 57(2), pp. 113–125.

Klevens, R.M., Fleming, P.L., Li, J., Gaines, C.G., Gallagher, K., Schwarcz, S., Karon, J., and Ward, J.W. (2001). The completeness, validity, and timeliness of AIDS surveillance data. *Annals of Epidemiology* 11, pp. 443–449.

Kozel, N.J. (1993). The Role of Networks in Drug Abuse Surveillance: An Account of the History, Implementation, and Development of the Community Epidemiology Work Group. In: *Health Related Data and Epidemiology in the European Community*, Commission of the European Communities, Office for Official Publications of the European Communities, L-2985 Luxembourg, pp. 37–57.

Lloyd-Jones, D.M., Wang, T.J., Leip, E.P., Larson, M.G., Levy, D., Vasan, R.S., D'Agostino, R.B., Massaro, J.M., Beiser, A., Wolf, P.A., and Benjamin, E.J. (2004). Lifetime risk for development of atrial fibrillation: The Framingham Heart Study. *Circulation* 110(9), pp. 1042–1046.

Medina-Mora, M.E., Cravioto, P., Ortiz, A., Kuri, P., and Villatoro, J. (2003). *Bulletin on Narcotics* LV(1 and 2), pp. 105–120.

National Cancer Institute website for the Surveillance, Epidemiology, and End Results: http://seer.cancer.gov.

National Heart, Lung, and Blood Institute website for the Framingham Heart Study: http://www.nhlbi.nih.gov/resources/deca/descriptions/framcohrt.htm.

National Institute on Drug Abuse. (1998). *Assessing Drug Abuse Within and Across Communities*, National Institutes of Health, NIH Publication No. 98-3614, Bethesda, Maryland.

National Institute on Drug Abuse. (1999). Epidemiological Trends in Drug Abuse—Volume II: Proceedings of the Community Epidemiology Work Group, December 1998, National Institutes of Health, NIH Publication No. 99-4527, Rockville, Maryland.

Nurco, D.N., Shaffer, J.W., Ball, J.C., and Kinlock, T.W. (1984). Trends in the commission of crime among narcotic addicts over successive periods of addiction and nonaddiction. American Journal of Drug and Alcohol Abuse 10(4), pp. 481–489.

Nurco, D.N., Kinlock, T.W., Hanlon, T.E., and Ball, J.C. (1988). Nonnarcotic drug use over an addiction career—a study of heroin addicts in Baltimore and New York City. Comprehensive Psychiatry 29(5), pp. 450–459.

Pach, A. and Gorman, E.M. (2003). An ethno-epidemiological approach for the multi-site study of emerging drug trends: the spread of methamphetamine in the United States of America. *Bulletin on Narcotics* LIV (1 and 2), pp. 87–102.

Price, R.K., Risk, N.K., and Spitznagel, E.L. (2001). Remission from drug abuse over a 25-year period: patterns of remission and treatment use. *American Journal of Public Health* 91(7), pp. 1107–1113.

Reynolds, G.l., Fisher, D.G., Wood, M.M., Klahn, J.A., and Johnson, M.E. (2003). Use of emergency room services by out-of-treatment drug users in Long Beach, California. *Journal of Addictive Diseases* 22(2), pp. 1–13.

Shai, D. (1994). Problems of accuracy in official statistics on drug-related deaths. *International Journal of the Addictions* 29(4), pp. 1801–1811.

Sloboda, Z. and Kozel, N.J. (2003). Understanding drug trends in the United States of America: the role of the Community Epidemiology Work Group as part of a comprehensive drug information system. *Bulletin on Narcotics* LV(1 and 2), pp. 41–52.

Smith Sehdey, A.E. and Hutchins, G.M. (2001). Problems with proper completion and accuracy of the cause-of-death statement. *Archives of Internal Medicine* 161(2), pp. 277–284.

Sterk, C.E. and Elifson, K W. (2005). Qualitative methods in the drug abuse field. In Sloboda, Z. (Ed.), *Epidemiology of Drug Abuse*. Kluwer Academic/Plenum Publishers, New York.

Substance Abuse and Mental Health Services Administration, Office of Applied Studies. (2003). *National Survey of Substance Abuse Treatment Services (N-SSATS): 2002. Data on Substance Abuse Treatment Facilities*, DASIS Series: S-19, DHHS Publication No. (SMA) 03–3777, Rockville, MD.

World Health Organization. (2000). *Guide to Drug Abuse Epidemiology*. WHO Publication, Geneva.

6

Sampling Issues in Drug Epidemiology

Colin Taylor and Paul Griffiths

COLIN TAYLOR AND PAUL GRIFFITHS • European Monitoring Centre on Drugs and Drug Addiction (EMCDDA)

1. INTRODUCTION

"A sample is a group of subjects selected from a larger group in the hope that studying this smaller group (the sample) will reveal important things about the larger group (the population)." This definition, taken from the 'Dictionary of statistics and methodology: a non-technical guide for the social sciences.' (Vogt 1993) highlights the central issue for sampling: that researchers study a small, known group but in general want to find out about an unknown, larger population. To support the hope that such inferences can be made, drug epidemiologists are faced with the same statistical and technical issues in the selection of the smaller group from the larger as researchers in other areas of social investigation, but unlike many other areas they are faced with a number of additional specific challenges that arise from the very nature of illicit drug use.

At one end of its spectrum illicit drug use is a covert and stigmatized behavior, and the other end of the spectrum, reaches into social acceptability and even common practice. Injecting drug users and opiate or crack-cocaine users are often termed a 'hidden population' or a 'hard-to-access' population, i.e., not only can they be relatively rare in general population terms and unwilling to participate in, or even hostile to, research activities, but as an identifiable group they are not readily accessed through administrative records. The concern of this chapter is to describe the issues of sampling this harder to reach end of the spectrum, working with the sub-group of known drug users who are at any one time in contact with, or come to the attention of, some sort of official body. At the 'softer' end, cannabis users by contrast are a less marginalized, relatively prevalent and more accessible group; in socially accepting settings, they may be more easily studied using more traditional survey techniques, especially when using methods that have been developed to help reduce both response and non-response biases.

The chapter considers how standard sample selection methods have been adapted and developed to overcome the difficulties that hard drug use presents. Sampling methods are usually designed to help with the quantification of behaviors; i.e., they aim to allow descriptions by counts and percentages to be meaningful, and the concerns here are principally with inferences in quantitative research methods. But the circumstances in which quantification is possible are often limiting and much of the research moves beyond aiming to quantify responses or characteristics in a population to more qualitative research approaches that do not usually attempt to make any statistically based inferences from their observations to the larger population. We note though that these same sampling procedures will often also benefit qualitative research that looks to generalize beyond its immediate subjects.

2. MOVING FROM STANDARD TO MORE INNOVATIVE SAMPLE SELECTION PROCEDURES

Prevalence estimation is one major area of interest for drug abuse researchers, but many studies need to access samples of drug users to explore numerous other topics such as the natural history and career of drug using, help seeking behavior, and the relationship of drug use to offending and to the development of health or social problems. In doing so, innovative adaptations to traditional random sampling procedures are required to overcome the difficulties inherent in selecting samples from this population group.

To understand how these techniques differ, three traditionally standard steps are underscored that enable a researcher to study scientifically the epidemiology, etiology and other characteristics of a disease, or of any behavior in the target population from which the observed sample group is drawn. These steps are crucial to traditional sampling methods because they can improve the chances that the sample selected for observation is representative of the target population and, while they cannot guarantee representativeness, they will allow the researcher to quantify how likely the sample is to be representative on any specified characteristic. Taken together, these steps form strong controls on the traditional selection procedures:

1. Define the target population and construct a list that includes all its members—sometimes this list can be constructed dynamically (as in multi-stage sampling, described below).
2. Select members from the complete list in a controlled, probabilistic way—while equal probability selections may be made, techniques may be necessary that stratify or boost differentially the selection, particularly if there are not many target individuals on the list, but the probability of selection from the list must remain known.
3. Find and interview the sample members, eliciting responses carefully using appropriate tools, measures and procedures—if not possible to interview them discreetly and confidentially in person, alternative ways of collecting the information can be used.

3. DEFINITIONS ARE DIFFICULT

The question of how to define the target population is probably more complex in the drug addiction field than in many others, as discussed more fully in Chapter 1.

It needs to be emphasized that the question of being a 'current drug user' is not the same sort of question as being 'HIV positive' for example, or as having some specific medical diagnosis. While these sorts of questions are not unique to drug abuse epidemiology, answering them does constitute a major task in a well designed study (e.g., Buster et al., 2001). While diagnostic criteria that apply to drug abuse and dependence have been developed under both the International Classification of Diseases 10 and the Diagnostic and Statistical Manual IV, these are often difficult to apply in many research settings in order to define target populations (e.g., Cottler et al., 2001). Usually studies use definitions based on simple behavioral measures of use of some specified drug type over time, with life-time prevalence (ever-use), last month prevalence, and days used in the last month being the most commonly used constructs.

Typically, studies focus on sub-groups of the overall general population, and target definition becomes crucial. For example, for the European Union a target group definition of drug use based on lifetime prevalence of any controlled substance would imply a target between 20 percent and 25 percent of the adult population, whereas a target population defined as current drug injectors would represent probably under 0.5 percent of the adult population of Europe. (EMCDDA, 2003)

Age restrictions are common in drug studies and are relatively easy to apply. As drug-taking behavior is most prevalent in the 15–35 age group, studies may focus exclusively on this range in order to conserve resources. Although drug use may be important outside this age range, studying it across its full age spread would be resource-intensive, making age-group definitions an important design factor.

A common feature of many drug studies is an emphasis on local populations. Drug-taking is often more prevalent and more easily studied in cities, for example, than at a national level. Using a local population presents definitional difficulties that need to be addressed carefully. For instance, determining what is a sensibly defined prevalence rate in a city might dramatically change as a result of broadening the definition of 'city limits'. Where people live is a question that is relatively easy to document if they have a permanent address but many drug users do not. Whether to include those who work or are receiving drug abuse treatment in the designated area, even if they live elsewhere, are issues that need to be given consideration and definitional precision, as these decisions can have a considerable effect on the overall size and the characteristics of the chosen target population.

4. GENERAL POPULATION SAMPLING FRAMES ARE OFTEN NOT USEFUL

Traditional survey methods for estimating levels of any behavior in a population, i.e., population or household surveys, are the standard ways for measuring prevalence. Indeed they can be very effective in monitoring the use of common and legal substances such as tobacco and alcohol, and to some extent cannabis. They are ineffective, however, at measuring the prevalence of rare, more covert, more stigmatized and more problematic forms of drug use such as injecting heroin or crack-cocaine use. There are numerous ways in which sampling bias can occur in this arena. For instance, injecting drug users or crack-cocaine users are less likely than non-problematic drug users to live in households that are included in general household surveys, injectors and crack-cocaine users may be less likely to agree to be surveyed if asked, and injecting may be less likely to be reported than other forms of drug use practices.

In addition to potential bias, further complications arise from the low prevalence of problem drug use within general population sampling frames, since any sample drawn will often identify so few users that reports of current injecting behaviors may be all but non-existent. Whether higher prevalence rates mean that other drug use, such as the use of cocaine (powder) or ecstasy, could be the subject of general surveys is a moot point (e.g. Degenhardt et al., in press). Survey data in both the United States and Europe show changes in use over time similar to information derived from indirect indicators of drug use (such as seizures and treatment demand). However the extent to which survey data directly reflects underlying trends for these substances remains unclear and other factors, such as changing social attitudes to drug use, also may be important. Survey techniques, such as the use of booster samples, have been developed to increase the numbers of drug users recruited into the sample. Chapter 7 reviews how survey techniques themselves have been adapted to deal with these difficulties. Nonetheless, for researchers wanting to study the behavior of those consuming drugs like heroin or crack cocaine or who are injecting drug users, a general population sampling frame as a starting point is not likely to be either a practical or a methodologically sound option.

4.1.   The Usefulness of Schools Surveys

One example of using a restricted sampling frame with definitional difficulties that is worthy of special note is schools surveys. Schools surveys are widely used for exploring exposure to drug use at a specific age or grade level and represent a valuable tool for tracking trends in exposure to drug use over time. School surveys though do have the same limitations as population surveys in respect of hard drug use. As a rule, to take account of the setting for the data collection, specially designed multi-stage cluster samples are used. In essence it is difficult to do other than collect a complete 'classroom-full of data' rather than to sample on an individual basis (UNODC, 2003). Furthermore, the sampling frame used in a multi-stage procedure can be simplified, in that listings of the classes that could be chosen need only be made for selected schools. For more information on school surveys refer to the European School Project on Alcohol and Drugs (Hibbell et al.,

2000), Monitoring the Future (Johnston et al., 2004), and to the Health Behavior in School-Aged Children (Currie et al., 2004).

4.2. Using Non-Standard Sampling Frames

School surveys, as described above, are one example of using (as in many two-stage sample surveys) dynamic sampling frame lists, i.e., lists that are never constructed in entirety but only in parts, as needed, in this case in a hierarchic fashion. Dynamic list construction is frequently used in drug abuse studies.

A close parallel to dynamic list construction is the use of area (quadrat) samples and line transect samples. The underlying principle of these approaches is using the physical, geographic layout of the population as a 'sampling frame', selecting clusters of people for the sample through their physical location rather than through a list. Such methods differ from more standard ones only in that the researcher does not know what fraction of the population is obtained in the sample, but in preserves the same statistical properties as those of a standard multi-stage or cluster sample. This method is particularly useful in countries or regions of a country where administrative records are poor or inadequate for compiling a complete sampling frame in the usual manner. This method, discussed more fully below, emerges in drug abuse epidemiology as 'site sampling' and is a major contributor to the development of sampling methods (McKeganey et al., 1992).

5. INFERENCES, SAMPLING CONTROL, BIASES AND ERRORS

One of the principal functions of using a comprehensive sampling frame in classical statistical probability sampling is to enable the researcher to have control over who enters and does not enter the sample. This may sound paradoxical, since the point is to obtain a *randomly derived* sample of the target population, but in fact this is achieved by selecting according to careful probability-based procedures. It should be emphatically distinguished from a *haphazard sample* into which entry is left to chance factors with no control. In such a sample there are always openings for large potential biases to occur, unknown to the researcher, under the whims of fate, other people, and other unidentified factors that determine what type of person is sampled. For instance, these factors may vary from a bias towards people who are available on a Tuesday afternoon (or whenever selection is carried out), who may be of a cheerful and pleasant disposition or of a compliant personality, and so forth. With a controlled sample selection, there is no causal connection between an individual's characteristics and whether or not that person is in or out of the sample; selection depends instead on the toss of a coin, for example, or some other random procedure.

The benefits that flow from probability sampling concern the degree to which the final sample is representative of the target population, focusing on measuring potential "unrepresentativeness." Indeed the whole point of statistical inference, estimation, reliability and confidence intervals can be regarded as quantifying how likely and to what degree the sample is representative of the target population, and using a known probabilistic random sampling procedure is central to these probability calculations.

5.1.   What Can Be Done with Non-Probabilistic Samples?

There are two types of non-probabilistic samples that have been commonly used for studying drug users because of their ease of implementation and the apparent directness of their sampling approach. The first type comes under a broad heading of 'convenience samples'. These samples are not constructed using probabilistic representation of the target population, but simply from convenience of access. This might mean the selection of a group of users who are at hand when the research is being planned or carried out or it may mean interviewing any of the researcher's contacts who are known to exhibit the target behavior. Whatever the access route, these samples provide almost no possibility of making broader inferences beyond those individuals immediately studied. These types of samples or study groups fall outside the scope of standard statistical analysis and inference because their ascertainment does not allow the usual generalizations from any analysis of them. These groups could possibly be classified under a heading of 'special populations' and useful insights have been gained from studying them in an explorative context.

The second type of non-probabilistic sample that offers more surface plausibility is one that is self-selected, i.e., the researcher's control over who enters the sample is relinquished and instead people who volunteer are used as a sample. A common procedure to recruit such a group is to advertise in a magazine, on a radio program, or through clubs that are known to have a high percentage of drug users among their readership, audience or clientele. Using this method of recruitment presents a number of biases such as special personality traits, drug-taking behavior, or demographic characteristics that will dramatically influence the findings from such a sample (Winstock et al., 2001; Inciardi and Harrison, 2000). It can be argued that even using a properly constructed approach, respondents need to agree to be interviewed and can refuse to take part, and so in some sense are still considered volunteers. It is well accepted, however, that should such biases, as measured by the number of refusals or more generally the non-response rate, become significant the study results can be severely compromised. It is worth noting that in a survey using a probability sample, the non-response rate can usually be calculated and it is often possible to determine what type of individual is failing to respond, so that corrections can be made for any inherent bias in the statistical analyses.

A third type of sampling is often used in epidemiological experimental and quasi-experimental studies, where the researcher selects a study group of drug abusers that is not intended to represent a larger population but rather to contain individuals who highlight some important characteristic. Many drug studies fall under this category; for example, drug injectors may be recruited who attend a low threshold treatment center and their injecting practices may differ when compared with those who attend specialist out-patient centers. For the most part these studies employ some sort of randomization of a factor of interest, such as type of treatment administered and in a technical sense the role of randomization becomes central. It is not possible though to use results from these studies in wider epidemiological inferences if the study groups have not been properly sampled. The resulting study conclusions are not treated as estimates in a population, but only as comparisons within the study group.

Much of what is done in estimating prevalence of problem drug use and in drawing drug user samples for study is an attempt to approximate random sampling procedures in order to acquire some sort of representative sample of drug users beyond those in contact with services or known to the authorities. Site sampling and chain referral sampling techniques are two vital components in these methods. The field of drug abuse epidemiology is a mixture of, on the one hand, well-formed analyses on special sub-populations that are in themselves usually targeted primarily because they can be sampled randomly, and on the other hand, a set of procedures that try to approximate random sampling of broader populations that are of interest.

5.2. Statistical and Non-Statistical Inferences—Moving From Best to Next Best

The benefits of using random sampling procedures are that the researcher is able to generalize beyond the 'known observations' in the sample and make probabilistic inferences to the whole target population from which the sample has been drawn. While highly desirable, this statistical ideal is not always practically achievable for many important topics of interest. Therefore a second type of inference can be made based on common knowledge and common sense non-statistical grounds. Moving outside statistical inference in this way means that certainty and uncertainty and the extent to which reliance can be placed on the conclusions is not quantifiable, only arguable. These approaches are important in all fields of behavioral research, moving beyond epidemiological results into a more interpretive arena, where such inferences are frequently necessary; and the drug research arena is no exception.

Many important studies in the drug abuse field have provided useful evidence even when probabilistic inference to the larger population could not be shown. For example, in most circumstances drawing an adequate sampling frame of drug injectors may be difficult to achieve. Nonetheless, studies based on injectors recruited in streets and other settings have yielded useful information on issues such as injecting practices that have extremely important implications for public health policy. In the design of such studies, drug abuse researchers consider what possible biases may be generated within the sample and seek to employ sampling techniques that will limit these. In the analysis of data from such studies it is important to compare the findings with work from other studies (Hartnoll, 1997; Stimson et al., 1997) and what is known about the target population, and to remember that caution is needed when trying to infer from the study to the population as a whole (e.g., Topp et al., 2004).

6.   MAKING THE MOST OF INCOMPLETE LISTS OF DRUG ABUSERS

The construction of a sampling frame is dependent on having, or being able to construct, a list covering all the members of the target population. In the drug epidemiology field only lists that include problem drug users are readily available but none of these are in any way complete. The type of list typically used is generally drug treatment admissions or discharges, but other lists are available in many countries such as arrests that either identify the arrestee as a drug user or that indicate that the arrest was made for a drug use offence; rosters of people attending social service agencies who are identified as drug users; records from accident and emergency hospital clinics; records from infectious diseases clinics that may identify drug injectors; and, deaths registers that indicate drug-related deaths. There are many limitations associated with use of these lists as are outlined in Chapter 5.

Cross-sectional and longitudinal surveys of heroin users and injecting drug users show that substantial proportions enter treatment, use harm reduction services, get arrested and often imprisoned. For example, a survey of recent injecting drug users in London reported that about 80 percent had attended a syringe exchange; over half had been tested for HIV or HCV; 40 percent had been in treatment; and 20 percent had been in prison since they started injecting. However, it has been found that over the duration of the studies, the proportion of time spent in treatment or in prison or having any contact with any service may be small (e.g., Hser et al., 1992) and there are examples of subjects initiating and ceasing injecting without having experienced any service contact at all (McKeganey and Platt, 1993; Inciardi and Harrison, 2000).

6.1.   Specialist Prevalence Estimation Methods

Under-ascertainment in each of many lists is in fact the basis for indirect methods of prevalence estimation. Modeling the under-ascertainment in each data source and in combinations of data sources and making restrictive assumptions, allows under-ascertainment factors to be calculated for the various sources separately and together. These techniques are described under the headings of Capture-recapture and Multiplier methods, covered in Chapter 8. They are however useful only in estimating prevalence of problem drug use and even then, with some considerable error potential. The error potential lies in two principal areas: the methods are dependent on randomly sampling the drug abuser population or at least approximating this, and the adjustment factors; i.e., the ratio of the unknown population of drug users to the number actually known, are often large.

6.2.   Re-Defining the Study Population

Drug abuse researchers have adopted a simple solution to the problem of incomplete ascertainment of the study population by re-defining the study population into one that *can* be sampled and from which statistical inferences can made only to this population and not the population as a whole. Thus a study interested in the behavior of drug injectors might draw a sample of those attending low threshold drug treatment services. Any further inference that is then made from these findings to injectors not in contact with these services would not be supported by statistical procedures but only by "what is reasonable to presume . . . "

6.3.   The Where, When and Who of Site Sampling

Sampling people without having a prior exhaustive sample frame but instead taking them from some physical or geographical sample point and if necessary at pre-specified times requires planning. A frequently used site sampling procedure in epidemiological studies is to sample at treatment centers, usually hospitals, for members of the target population. In more difficult circumstances an existing list may not be available and drug abuse epidemiologists must construct one as they go along. Many of the services that work with the most hard-to-reach drug users make it a policy not to collect information that identifies their clients whose attendance may be sporadic and brief. Sometimes samples are collected from known areas where drug users congregate and the task is to develop a sampling frame that reflects those drug users who visit this geographical space. TenHouten et al. (1971) discuss the idea of extending such site samples to a plurality of sites in order to sample more effectively from the whole population under study. Hendricks and colleagues (1992) describe an approach that sketches out a map of the city's likely congregation centers for cocaine use in order to draw a multi-site sample from these centers. Depending upon the frequency of occurrence at the sample points, sampling may be systematic, say every fifth identified individual; randomly selecting one fifth of the individuals in true binomial sampling fashion;

or by exhaustive sampling of all individuals within a given time span. Whichever the precise details, the selection procedure within a site needs controlled, careful execution using well-defined principles in the same way as when using a standard sampling frame.

The most common example in the drug abuse research literature of this sort of sampling approach is in treatment studies where, for example daytime attendees at a clinic, hospital or other center are recruited for the study and handled as a randomly sampled selection from the whole population, potential and actual. Note that in this example the population being studied may have been re-defined deliberately to accommodate the sampling procedure.

6.3.1. Site Coverage, Site Attendances and Weighted Sampling

There are two principal questions concerning site sampling: to what extent is the entire target population encompassed and how often do different individuals attend the site or sites. Drawing a random sample of sites is important in order to be able to make subsequent inferences from the sample to population. Any potential sampling scheme should be considered using some specified conceptual typing such as stratification by physical location so that randomization procedures can be applied within each stratum. Failure to achieve a random sample of sites means that any statistical inferences are restricted solely to the sites actually observed without the ability to generalize to the populations at other sites.

The second important issue related to site sampling that has received little attention in the literature is that unless all population members attend the site(s) in question with the same frequency, simple random sampling procedures cannot be used. If some types of drug abusers, attend twice as frequently as others, then in any given time-period of sampling that group will be twice as likely to be drawn into the sample. Site sampling over-samples subjects in direct proportion to the natural frequency of attendance at the site and it is therefore paramount that in site sampling every effort is made to identify the frequency of attendance of sample members at all the various sites that are being used in the sampling scheme and their weighting applied in subsequent analyses. For example, a study of injectors attending pharmacy-based needle and syringe provision in London required a sampling strategy accounting for the variation not only in the number of clients seen across pharmacies but also in the frequency by which injectors accessed them; some would attend daily picking up a small amount of supplies while others would appear only sporadically but take away enough supplies to last them for longer periods of time (Clarke et al., 2001). Failure to allow for this differential weighting will result in the analysis and description being made of *attendance* and not *attendees* at the clinic or site.

7.   MOVING INTO THE UNKNOWN—THE ROLE OF NOMINATION METHODS AND CHAIN REFERRALS

The concept of 'hard-to-access' populations has lead drug researchers to use a number of methods to move the immediate knowledge base beyond those drug abusers observed to the wider drug abusing population. In so doing, the intention is to use any available partial listing or dynamically constructed listing of drug abusers to give wider access to the target population. The two primary methods are both dependent on what are called 'nomination' techniques.

7.1.   Nomination Methods

Nomination methods are general estimation methods based on information that individuals in a sample provide about their network of acquaintances (e.g. Biernacki and Waldorf, 1981; Morrison 1988; Stimson et al. 1997). One instance of the application of nomination methods is in estimating drug abuse prevalence using benchmark/ratio methods that require an estimation of the proportion of drug users who are, for example, in treatment (e.g., Taylor, 1997). Simply put, a core sample of drug users recruited in an accessible setting is asked to name (nominate) their drug-using acquaintances and then to say whether these acquaintances have been in touch with any drug treatment centers, health services, or any other similar body within a stipulated time period. It is important when asking these questions that definitions of 'drug user' and 'treatment' are precise and that other qualifiers such as time and geographical location are clearly understood. From this information, the proportion of drug users in treatment can be calculated. This is an obvious adaptation from the more direct question: "What proportion of your drug-using acquaintances have been in treatment?" which is less useful as it is a more difficult question to answer and the answer itself may be subject to rounding off than when asked in two stages. Also, as the baseline number of drug users is not known, weighting each respondent's answer by its statistical reliability is not possible. Clearly there is a trade-off between having information on a greater number of drug users using the nomination technique at the expense of information accuracy. The respondents' personal impressions of the drug-using population and treatment are actually being recorded and the accuracy of the information will depend upon how well the respondent answers or can be encouraged to answer the two questions. It would be inadvisable to ask questions such as the precise frequency of poly-drug use or being tested for HIV as this information may not be known as reliably by respondents other than for themselves.

Nonetheless, the value of nomination methods is that they give the researcher the ability to extend information beyond the core sample of observed drug users to the unobserved population. Although the information so acquired is limited, it can be used to give indirect information on several aspects of drug users' behaviors.

From a sampling point of view, representativeness depends on the selection of the initial sample and, for reasons we have already discussed, this means at best that it is representative of some more restrictively defined population. Theoretical assessments of these methods have been slow but they broadly follow the tradition of two-stage cluster sampling and closely parallel 'star sampling' used in ecology (Thompson and Seber, 1996). Parker and colleagues (1987) offer one of the few comparisons of the impact of different nomination techniques in a study estimating the number of opiate users in four English towns.

7.2.   Following-Up the Nominations—The Chain Referral or Snowball Sample

A snowball or chain referral sample is an extension of nomination methods where the initial sample's (termed 'zero stage sample') nominees are traced, interviewed and in turn asked for further nominees. This process is then repeated for a number of further stages (e.g., Stimson et al., 1997). Although a snowball sample can begin at stage zero with sampling from an incomplete list of drug users, it is better to begin with some random site selection procedure. The purpose of this technique is to penetrate into networks of drug users that would be difficult and costly to reach by any other procedure. The value of the approach is confirmed by the long list of informative qualitative and quantitative studies that have used this method for sample generation. Drug use is a socially mediated behavior and drug users as a rule inhabit linked social networks that the snowball sampling procedure exploits.

7.2.1.   Snowballing Theory and Snowballing Practice

The following much-quoted key areas for snowball sampling were originally put forward by Biernacki and Waldorf (1981): i) finding respondents and starting referral chains; ii) verifying the eligibility of potential respondents; iii) engaging respondents as research assistants, iv) controlling the types of chains and number of cases, and, v) checking and monitoring referral chains and data quality. It is important to note that only two of these are concerned with the statistical theoretical aspects of snowball sampling and that the remainder deal with practical ground level considerations. This is reflected in the fact that many studies that use this approach have to a large extent ignored statistical sampling issues and have tended to be content with generating a large number of people who exhibit specific target behavior such as drug injecting. Exploratory studies use snowball sampling to penetrate networks of drug users as there are few alternative methods available.

Rapoport (1979; 1980) among others has theoretically reviewed the idea of penetration into social networks. The concerns then shift from whether the sample is randomly drawn to whether representativeness in some sense can be achieved through other controls and to what extent the link tracing can give access to the whole of a specific network. Mathematical analysis of what are called 'biased net-works' has managed to progress only through making unrealistic assumptions that give the crudest practical guide to the researcher. In practice, different link-tracing rules, different drugs, and different social strata, all create different problems that need to be addressed in a research design in the absence of detailed, theoretical guidance from the probability sampling perspective. It would seem possible, for example, that heroin-using networks might be more closely knit than cocaine-using networks, that middle-class drug users might be less prepared to nominate drug-using acquaintances, and that treatment centers will give better access to opi-ate users than to cocaine users. In these circumstances the only consensus advice appears to be that the initial sample is at least spread as widely as possible across the target population and is as large as possible. It would also seem useful to pursue chains to their full length (sampling to extinction) wherever this is possible.

Snowball samples of this sort can be useful in a number of ways (e.g., Trotter and Medina-Mora, 2000; Fountain et al. 2000). Determining the range of types of behavior patterns or types of individuals is possible by using classification (or cluster) analysis methods that do not need to account for the frequency with which the behavior types occur. Relationships between variables are sometimes more robust than is prevalence to non-representativeness. Modeling the relationship of a particular response (for instance the presence of HIV) to other variables (such as age or injection practices) does not necessarily require accurate representation on these explanatory variables; it requires a sample that does not preferentially contact say HIV cases among young groups. How far a non-random sample can be nearly-representative is influenced by a great variety of factors, amongst them the number of initial recruits, the extent to which contacts form into closed cliques, and the extent to which cliques are connected. Generalization from such a sample to the whole population must be made without the benefit of statistical confidence calculations.

But not all studies have taken this restrictive approach. Others have attempted to build random selection procedures into their sampling, although the theoretical basis for the procedures is often unclear (Bieleman et al., 1993). Goodman (1961) has developed mathematical models that provide statistically valid estimates for the population from a chain referral sample. In practice this means the potential benefits that can come from adopting procedures that statistically underpin the sample have to be balanced against those that generate a large sample and can be accomplished in practice.

That said, many of the methodological and practical difficulties of generating a snowball sample are unrelated to statistical issues. For example, interviewer selection is extremely important, as most successful snowball sampling designs require the contact and interview of drug abusers in naturalistic settings. Some studies have taken this issue further by using members of the target community as interviewers with apparent success in generating sample numbers, particularly groups that are in some respect closed to outsiders such as drug users from ethnic minority populations. As with all referral techniques, attention to ethical and health and safety issues is of paramount importance. The following references discuss these methods in more depth; Fountain, 2004, Griffiths et al., 1993, and Power and Harkinson, 1993.

7.2.2. Using Chain Referrals in a Sampling Procedure

From a sampling point of view the purpose of the study; be it exploratory, descriptive and modeling or attempting to draw inference about the population, will determine the way the snowball sample is constructed. In defining a chain referral sampling procedure three factors are important: the method for recruiting the zero wave sample, the number of waves (link tracing procedures) the sample uses, and the rules that are used to make nominations.

7.2.2.1. Recruitment. There are no formal theoretical statistical guidelines on what type of zero wave procedure to adopt save only that if a snowball sample is to have any technical statistical validity in making inference to a larger population it must begin with a seeding sample that is randomly drawn and as large as possible. This can be difficult to achieve in practice although the introduction of site sampling in the absence of a population sampling frame has enabled snowball sampling theory to develop along classical statistical lines. Using this combined sampling model has been a major step forward in theoretical terms. If the initiating site sample can be constructed as a probability sample, statistical inferences can be made to the population from both the zero stage sample and from the complete snowball sample. TenHouten et al. (1971) incorporated the two sampling methods, site sampling and snowball sampling, in their analysis of a community's leadership structure.

Snowball samples even if not generated by an initial random sample may still be useful for some other purposes. In these circumstances it is probably advisable to make sure the initial sample is at least spread across the conceived target population as much as possible and it is often recommended that in this first wave all available nominee links be traced.

7.2.2.2. Waves. There is a variety of ways to determine the number of waves of nominee follow-up in a snowball sample. The first and foremost issue is whether they are fixed to be the same for every chain generated by the sample or are allowed to vary naturally as nominations proceed. In spite of ground-breaking work by Goodman (1961), the theoretical consequences even for approximating statistical inferences about population parameters are not clear particularly in terms of efficient use of a given sample size or collection effort or in terms of the degree to which the resulting estimates are unbiased.

For most purposes it would seem inefficient to fix the number of stages in advance. Usually the primary consideration is to obtain enough people by the procedure to allow reasonable numbers for analysis or description. It seems preferable for efficient administrative effort to let the nomination process proceed without imposing constraints on its format. The procedure can be terminated either by sampling to extinction; i.e., until the last wave adds no new nominees or by reaching a pre-determined number of sample members.

7.2.2.3. Nomination Rules. In terms of practical fieldwork, organizing the number of links for selecting nominees at each stage in a snowball procedure is easiest when a uniform set of rules is used for each sample member rather than allowing them to vary haphazardly as the sample waves progress. For any given set of rules, however, Hendricks et al. (1992) note that the theoretical implications are unclear and the best choice might depend rather upon the goal of the study. Each study has different purposes and has both advantages and disadvantages in terms of rate of growth of the sample, costs, and risks of a restricted or biased sample. They provide speculative guidelines which evidence good common sense; for example, tracing all links nominated by the respondent should allow for rapid growth, whereas, tracing links drawn at random may help reduce some concerns about potential biases by maintaining a constant randomization factor in each nomination step. Some work has looked at tracing links in a pre-determined order of importance from the list of the respondent's nominees, taking either a fixed number from or a fixed proportion of the list. For example use of "*first best friend*" and "*second best friend*" and so on may allow for lines of closest or more distant contact to be followed up. Tracing links in a pre-determined reverse importance order (or "*least well known*", "*second* least *well known*" etc) from the list of the respondent's nominees may also produce a well-balanced sample. Although this is perhaps difficult to implement in practice, Rapoport observed (1979) that a tracing through "loose ties" between nominators and nominees will yield a spread sample similar to that derived from a completely randomized network model.

8.   CONCLUDING REMARKS AND RECOMMENDATIONS FOR GOOD PRACTICE

As any quantitative drug abuse researcher will point out, talking to even a small number of drug users can produce a wealth of information for understanding behavior that often challenges commonly held beliefs about drug use. For this reason, researchers have been content to dispense with the benefits offered by probability sampling theory and opt for any method that allows them access to sufficient numbers of drug users who exhibit the particular aspect of the behavior of interest. For many purposes the samples that are produced by conventional methods simply do not produce sufficient numbers for any meaningful analysis or may even exclude those who are often of most interest. Drug studies are sometimes criticized by those naïve to the issues of this area for their lack of sampling rigor, when often in practice less insight would have been achieved by adopting a conventional approach to sample generation.

That said, drug abuse epidemiology has attempted to exploit the analytical benefits from sampling theory, the major driving forces being the attempt to deal with the absence of a sampling frame, working with ambiguous definitions, and encompassing a broad range of behaviors and a correspondingly broad range of research needs. As far as possible conventional survey techniques have been adapted to take into account difficulties of accessing drug users and important study groups such as the school population. But all research studies are faced with the fact that to date all statistically valid estimation techniques require an initial random sample of the hidden population that has been defined as the target population. All the methods discussed above are framed by this requirement and are based on attempting to define the study population in some way that allows a valid sampling frame to be produced or at least approximated.

The easiest way to remain within the boundaries of conventional sampling approaches, at least in theory, is to define the population in such a way that a list can be produced, such as drug users attending treatment facilities, needle exchanges, or other low threshold services. Valuable information has been generated by such studies but statistical inference about drug users not in contact with these services is not possible.

Site sampling approaches, i.e., randomly sampling individuals within randomly selected sites and attempting to correct for variation in frequency of appearance at these sites, provides a solution to the problem if properly carried out. Site sampling can also help supply initial random sampling of the hidden population required by nomination methods and chain referral sampling, where a larger, better initial stage mitigates the clustering effects likely in later stages. It should be noted though that this implies defining the target population as the drug users who will inhabit the space the sites cover and drug users who do not are still excluded. Although they represent an import step forward in theory, it is both practically and methodologically difficult to construct such samples and properly drawn random samples of the general drug-abusing population, which are hidden or are otherwise inaccessible, are simply often not achievable in practice. Other methods are by default the only avenues of potential development in many areas with snowball techniques being the only practical way of generating a sample from many important populations. Furthermore, if nearly-representative samples can be achieved they can be useful in determining the range and pattern of relationships in hidden populations through classification analysis and modeling techniques.

Not all studies require representativeness of the whole drug using population or even the target population. Analysis of within sample differences can be useful and important policy inferences may not necessarily require statistical underpinning, even if desirable. For example, if a large chain referral sample of drug injectors shows that many are homeless and that high risk injecting practices are commonplace, then this information can be sufficient for prompting policy responses even if it is not possible to statistically quantify these behaviors in the total injecting population. Obviously, such analysis must be made with caution and one would want to be assured that recruitment methods avoided biases wherever possible, especially biases toward homelessness or high-risk behavior. In conclusion then drug researchers are faced with a complex set of practical, methodological and theoretical issues to balance in their research designs. Only some of these are related to sampling but the benefits that probabilistic sampling procedures can bring are sometimes simply unobtainable or have a restrictive impact on the topics for subsequent analysis. A consideration of sampling issues though is still a critical component in any investigation in this area. Drug abuse researchers need to continue to strive to employ probability methods where they can, make a best approximation where this is impossible, always be mindful of the importance of target population definition, and be aware how in practice this may differ from the intended group of drug users who are of interest. Most importantly, caution and sensitivity to possible biases should be used when making inferences from information that does not have the benefit of being based on probability techniques and collaborative evidence should be sought wherever possible.

REFERENCES

Bieleman, B., Diaz, A., Merlo, G., and Kaplan Ch.D. (1993). *Lines across Europe: nature and extent of cocaine use in Barcelona, Rotterdam and Turin.* Svets and Zeitlinger, Amsterdam.

Biernacki, P. and Waldorf, D. (1981). Snowball sampling: Problems and techniques of chain referral sampling. *Sociological Methods and Research* 10 (2), pp. 141–163.

Buster, M.C.A., van Brussel, G.H.A., and van de Brink, W. (2001). Estimating the number of opiate users in Amsterdam by capture-recapture: The importance of case definition. *European Journal of Epidemiology* 17, pp. 935–942.

Clarke, K., Sheridan, J., Griffiths, P., Noble, N., Williamson, S., and Taylor. C. (2001). Pharmacy needle exchange: do clients and community pharmacists have matching perceptions? *Pharmaceutical Journal* 266, pp. 553–556.

Cottler et al., 2001. L. Cottler, S.B. Womack, W.M. Compton and A. Ben-Abdallah, Ecstasy abuse and dependence among adolescents and young adults: applicability and reliability of DSM-IV criteria. *Hum. Psychopharmacol.: Clin. Exp.* 16 (2001), pp. 599–606.

Currie, C., Roberts, C., Morgan, A. et. al. (2004). *Young People's Health in Context. Health Behaviour in School Aged Children (HBSC) Study, International Report From The 2001/2002 Survey, Health Policy for Children and Adolescents*, No 4, World Health Organization, Geneva.

Degenhardt et al., in press. Degenhardt, L., Barker, B., Topp, L., in press. Ecstasy use in Australia: findings from a general population survey. Addiction.

European Monitoring Centre for Drugs and Drug Addiction. (2003). *Annual Report 2003: The State of the Drug Problem in the European Union and Norway*. European Monitoring Centre for Drugs and Drug Addiction, Lisbon.

Fountain, J. (Ed). (2004). *Young Refugees and Asylum Seekers in Greater London: Vulnerability to Problematic Drug Use.* Greater London Alcohol and Drug Alliance, Greater London Authority, London.

Fountain, J., Hartnoll, H., Olszewski, D., and Vicente J. (2000). (Eds.), *Understanding and Responding to Drug Use: The Role of Qualitative Research.* EMCDDA Scientific Monograph Series No. 4., EMCDDA, Lisbon.

Goodman, L.A. (1961). Snowball sampling. *Annals of Mathematical Statistics* 32, pp. 148–170.

Griffiths, P., Gossop, M., Powis, B., and Strang, J. (1993). Reaching populations of drug users by the use of privileged access interviewers: methodological and practical issues. *Addiction* 88, pp. 1617–1626.

Hartnoll R. (1997). Estimating the Prevalence of Problem Drug use in Europe. In: Stimson G.V., Hickman M., Quirk A., Frischer M. and Taylor C. (Eds.), *EMCDDA Scientific Monograph Series (No. 1).* Office for Official Publications of the European Communities, Luxemburg.

Hendricks, V.M., Blanken, P., and Adriaans, N.F.P. (1992). *Snowball Sampling: A Pilot Study on Cocaine Use.* IVO, Rotterdam.

Hibell, B., Andersson, B., Ahlstrom, S. et al. (2000). *The 1999 ESPAD Report: The European School Survey Project on Alcohol and Other Drugs.* The Swedish Council for Information on Alcohol and other drugs (CAN) and Council of Europe Pompidou Group.

Hser, Y., Anglin, M.D., Wickens, T.D., Brecht, M.L., and Homer J. (1992). *Techniques for the Estimation of Illicit Drug User Prevalence: An Overview of Relevant Issues.* National Institute of Justice, Washington, D.C.

Inciardi, J. and Harrison, L. (Eds.) (2000), *Harm Reduction: National and International Perspectives.* Sage Publications, Thousand Oaks, CA.

Johnston, L.D., O'Malley, P.M., Bachman, J.G., and Schulenberg, J.E. (2004). *Monitoring The Future National Survey Results on Drug Use, 1975–2003. Volume I: Secondary School Students.* National Institute on Drug Abuse, Bethesda, MD.

McKeganey N. Barnard M. Leyland A. Coote I., and Follet E. (1992). Female street-working prostitution and HIV infection in Glasgow. *British Medical Journal* 305, pp. 801–804.

McKeganey, N. and Platt, S. (1993). Estimating the population prevalence of injection drug use and infection with human immunodeficiency virus among injection drug users in Glasgow, Scotland. *American Journal of Epidemiology*, 138 (3), pp. 170–181.

Parker, H., Newcombe, R., and Bakx K. (1987). The new heroin users: prevalence and characteristics in Wirral, Merseyside. *British Journal of Addiction* 82, p. 4757.

Power, R. and Harkinson, S. (1993). Accessing hidden populations: A survey of indigenous interviewers. In Davies, P., Hart, G., and Aggleton, P. (Eds.), *Social aspects of AIDS.* Falmer Press, New York. pp. 109–119.

Rapoport, A. (1979). Some problems relating to randomly constructed biased networks. In Holland, P.W. and Leinhardt, S. (Eds.), *Perspectives on Social Network Research.* Academic Press, New York. pp. 119–136.

Rapoport, A. (1980). A probabilistic approach to networks. *Social Networks* 2, pp. 1–18.

Stimson, G.V., Hickman, M., Quirk, A., Frischer, M., and Taylor C. (Eds.), (1997). *Estimating the Prevalence of Problem Drug use in Europe. EMCDDA Scientific Monograph Series (No. 1).* Office for Official Publications of the European Communities, Luxemburg.

Taylor, C. (1997). Introduction to multiplier methods. In: Stimson, G., Hickman M., Quirk A. and Frischer M. (Eds.), *Estimating the Prevalence of Drug Misuse in Europe.* Council of Europe, Strasbourg, pp. 111–112.

TenHouten, W.D., Stern, J., and TenHouten D. (1971). Political Leadership in Poor Communities: Applications of Two Sampling Methodologies. In: Orleans, P. and Ellis Jr., W.R. *Race, Change and Urban Society*, Vol 5, Urban Affairs Annual Review, Sage Publications, Beverly Hills, CA.

Thompson, S.K. And Seber, G.A.F. (1996). *Adaptive Sampling.* John Wiley, New York.

Topp L., Degenhardt L., and Barker B. (2004). The external validity of results derived from ecstasy users recruited using purposive sampling strategies. Drug and Alcohol Dependence, Volume 73, Issue 1, 7 January 2004, pp. 33–40m in Science Direct.

Trotter, R. and Medina-Mora, M-E. (2000). In: *Guide to Drug Abuse Epidemiology.* WHO/MSD/MSB 00.3, World Health Organization, Geneva.

United Nations Office of Drugs and Crime. (2003). *Global Assessment Programme on Drug Abuse (GAP) Toolkit Module 3 Conducting School Surveys on Drug Abuse.* United Nations Office on Drugs and Crime, Vienna.

Vogt, W.P. (1999). *Dictionary of Statistics and Methodology: A Non-Technical Guide for the Social Sciences.* Sage Publications, Thousand Oaks, CA.

Winstock, A.R., Griffiths, P., and Stewart, D. (2001). Drugs and the dance music scene: A survey of current drug use patterns among a sample of dance music enthusiasts in the UK. *Drug and Alcohol Dependence* 64(1), pp. 9–17.

7

Collecting Drug Use Data from Different Populations

Edward M. Adlaf

1. INTRODUCTION

The primary goal of surveys investigating drug use behavior is to obtain valid and accurate measures of drug use that contribute to our knowledge, and, in turn, can be used to inform policy. Whether this goal can be fully realized is partly based on the interplay among the sampling methods used, the mode of interview, and the nature of the population under study. This chapter reviews the current state of the application of survey data collection methods employed for various populations.

EDWARD M. ADLAF • Centre for Addiction and Mental Health, and Departments of Public Health Sciences and Psychiatry, University of Toronto

2.   GENERAL POPULATION SURVEYS

Drug use estimates derived from general population surveys are considered essential for surveillance programs (Griffiths and McKetin, 2003). The key strengths of general population surveys include (1) random probability sampling that allows for generalization to the population, (2) the use of samples to capture the largest segment of the total population, and (3) the ability to calculate errors. Although surveys are powerful epidemiologic tools, when applied to substance abuse, they are subject to potential errors because of (1) self-reported drug use, (2) nonresponse, and (3) the exclusion of various groups from the target population (e.g., homeless).

Summarizing the expansive literature on the collection of drug use data from general population surveys is a task that goes well beyond the scope of this chapter. Indeed, during the past twenty years, methodological studies on general population surveys have increased in both scope and sophistication. If there is a gold standard of general population surveys it would be the U.S. National Survey on Drug Use and Health (NSDUH), formerly the National Household Survey on Drug Abuse, sponsored by Substance Abuse and Mental Health Services Administration (Substance Abuse and Mental Health Services Administration, 2004). Using a multi-stage area probability sample, about 68,000 respondents aged 12 years and older are surveyed every year. Interviews are conducted in-person, using a combination of computer-assisted personal interviewing (CAPI) and audio computer-assisted self-interviewing (ACASI) for sensitive drug use questions. The methods employed in this survey are based on an on-going methodological program that has identified the need for self-administered questions (Turner et al., 1992).

The NSDUH, however, is a survey of such a large scope and necessary resources, that few countries or regions can emulate it. Indeed, international principles of data collection of drug use information argue that data sources should be not only timely and relevant, but feasible and cost-efficient for sponsors (Griffiths and McKetin, 2003). It is for this reason that data collection methods for general population surveys can vary widely within and among countries.

Many of the data collection issues related to substance use surveys have been driven by changing technological capabilities. One of the earlier developments was the growth in random digit dialing (RDD) telephone surveys. Given the important advantages of telephone surveys compared to in-house interviews, such as lower costs, lower sampling error, many on-going surveillance surveys now employ telephone methods as their mode of data collection (Centers for Disease Control and Prevention, 2004; Grulich et al., 2003; Hall et al., 1991; Kilpatrick et al., 2003; MacNeil and Webster, 1997; Midanik and Greenfield, 2003; Wallisch, 2001; Wilkins et al., 2003).

The earlier research literature comparing telephone to face-to-face methods suggested that telephone methods generally faired well (de Leeuw and van der

Zouwen, 1988; Groves et al., 2004). However, research on drug use self-reports during the 1980s and 1990s clearly showed that self-administered methods provided higher drug use reports compared to telephone interviews (Aquilino, 1992; Aquilino, 1994; Gfroerer and Hughes, 1992; Gfroerer and Hughes, 1991; Schober et al., 1992; Turner et al., 1992). Turner et al. (1992), for example, found that respondents were about 2.5 times more likely to report past month cocaine use in a self-administered format than by telephone. Also noteworthy, was that this mode difference declined as the reporting period increased to past year use and to lifetime use. These empirical studies have also shown that this mode difference is nominal or non-existent for drugs such as alcohol and cannabis. It is also important to note that several studies have not found such differences (de Leeuw and van der Zouwen, 1988; Mangione et al., 1982), and some have found higher drug use estimates in telephone interviews (Sykes and Collins, 1988).

Despite the limitations of telephone surveys, it is likely that they will continue to be employed, especially by addiction professionals and public health organizations that require cost-efficient, timely data. Moreover, some recent research suggests that reporting error in telephone surveys can be improved with the use of telephone audio computer-assisted self-interviewing (T-ACASI). In this method, a human interviewer screens eligible respondents, but then transfers the respondent to a computer-controlled, pre-recorded questions read to the respondent, who then provides responses by touch tone entry. Limited pilot studies suggest that such technologies improve the reporting of sensitive behaviors (Gribble et al., 2000; Turner et al., 1996).

3. SPECIAL POPULATION SURVEYS

3.1. School Surveys

Perhaps the most salient of the special population surveys is students. Indeed, student surveys have many important advantages, including (1) the relative ease of developing full-probability sampling methods, (2) the cost-efficiency of school-based sampling, (3) good response rates, (4) the prevention importance among the adolescent population, (5) the anonymity of classroom administration, and (6) the cost efficiency is feasible for countries or regions that cannot afford a large general population survey (Griffiths and McKetin, 2003; Smart et al., 1980; United Nations Office on Drugs and Crime, 2003). These advantages explain the long history and dominance of school surveys in substance use epidemiology (Adlaf and Paglia, 2003; Centers for Disease Control and Prevention, 2004; Hibell et al., 2000; Johnston, O'Malley and Bachman, 2002; Smart and Ogborne, 2000). Yet, school surveys are not without their weaknesses, which include (1) the absence of dropouts from the target population, (2) non-respondent loss due to absent students,

(3) the increasing requirement for active parental consent forms, (4) the increasing difficulties in obtaining permission to survey students from school authorities, and (5) the underreporting of drug use by students (United Nations Office on Drugs and Crime, 2003).

Yet unlike general population surveys, mode variation is generally minimal in school surveys, with group-based self-administered questionnaires being the mode of choice. There are important reasons for this. First, individualized interviewing is costly and is seen as a complication for school authorities compared to classroom or group administration. Second, the empirical literature has consistently shown that school-based drug estimates are typically higher compared to other methods (Gfroerer, 1985; Gfroerer et al., 1997; Rootman and Smart, 1985; Sudman, 2001). The overwhelming basis for this finding is the perceived anonymity of self-administered questionnaires generally (Turner et al., 1992) and class-administration specifically (Gfroerer et al., 1997; O'Malley et al., 2000; Sudman, 2001).

Two issues are particular to student surveys—the impact of absent students and the loss due to consent form requirements. Although there is some research on these issues, given the frequent inability to incorporate full experimental control and the absence of strong theoretical models underlying survey participation in school surveys, we still lack an understanding of potential error caused by these sources. For example, although there is strong evidence that absent students differ from students that are present on the day of the survey, drug use differences between these two groups have been nominal or inconsistent (Guttmacher et al., 2002; Johnston and O'Malley, 1985).

The impact of consent form loss also complicates the character of potential bias in student surveys. Indeed, more and more Research Ethics Boards and school authorities are requiring the use of active parent consent forms (i.e., the student is allowed to participate only if the parent agrees in a signed consent form) than passive consent forms (i.e., the student is allowed to participate as long as the parent does not object) which were more commonly used in the past. The published literature in this area centers on three issues: the magnitude of the loss; the differential characteristics of students with and without consent; and the impact of consent loss on drug use estimates.

Assessing the overall magnitude of the loss due to parental consent, be it active or passive, is difficult given that many surveys do not report this loss (Hallfors and Iritani, 2002). The Ontario Student Drug Use Survey, for example, found that 16 percent of 7th- to 12th-graders in 2003 did not participate due to the absence of active parental consent, and that this percentage increased with increasing requirements of active parental consent, which averaged 4 percent between 1985 and 1991 (Adlaf and Paglia, 2003). It is also important to note that the impact of consent form loss is complex since it tends to interact with absenteeism. For example, while active parental consent form loss declined with grade, from 25 percent in grade 7 to 9 percent in grade 12, loss due to absent students increased from 7 percent in grade 7 to 19 percent in grade 12 (Adlaf and Paglia, 2003).

The research literature regarding the differential characteristics between active consent and passive consent samples has generally demonstrated notable differences suggesting that compared to passive consent samples, active consent samples have higher grades and fewer missed days of school (Henry et al., 2002), and are more likely to live with both parents, have a higher socio-economic status, and are more likely to be White (Dent et al., 1993).

Yet, despite these sample differences, research on the impact of consent form loss on drug use estimates is far from conclusive, given that some studies have found large differences in drug use between active consent and non-consent students, while others have found no differences (Dent et al., 1997; Severson and Ary, 1983). The literature does seem to suggest, however, that the impact of consent on drug use estimates is greater for younger students, and minimal for older students (Anderman et al., 1995; Dent et al., 1997; White et al., 2004).

In sum, the literature on the validity of drug use reported in school surveys indicates that, although self-reported drug use will underestimate the "true" usage, survey estimates have sufficient validity and reliability for epidemiological purposes (Brener et al., 2003; Johnson and Mott, 2001; Medina-Mora et al., 1981; O'Malley and Johnston, 2002; O'Malley et al., 2000).

Several challenges will face drug use researchers who work in the school setting. First, and foremost, will be to maintain response rates given increasing requirements of active parental consent forms, the need for independent Research Ethics approval by school authorities, and competing for limited class time. Some researchers have suggested that greater resources be used, such as greater school and parental contact, in order to increase consent form approval and response rates (Harrington et al., 1997; O'Donnell et al., 1997). As well, in 2003, the Monitoring the Future study began to pay participating schools as an incentive (Johnston et al., 2004). A second challenge will be to improve the data quality provided by participating students. Although there has been substantial research on the reliability and validity of self-reported drug use of students, we have yet to make significant gains in practice.

3.2. Campus Surveys

Another special population in the substance use area is college students. Although many campus surveys have a strong focus on heavy drinking, many also provide epidemiological estimates of drug use. (Abdullah et al., 2002; Adlaf et al., 2003; Bell et al., 1997; Kerber and Wallisch, 1999; Mangweth et al., 1997; Martinez et al., 1999; Meilman et al., 1990; Mohler-Kuo et al., 2003; O'Malley and Johnston, 2002; Pope et al., 2001; Prendergast, 1994; Strote et al., 2002; Webb, 1996).

Dedicated validity studies of self-reported drug use in this population are generally fewer compared to elementary and secondary school students, where experimental manipulation is easier. Moreover, as O'Malley and Johnston (2002) have argued, the extensive literature indicating the practical utility of self-reports should hold for university as well as younger students.

In the college population, the dominant mode of data collection has been self-administered mail questionnaires (e.g., Gliksman et al., 2000; Mohler-Kuo et al., 2003). The strengths of this method include the following: (1) self-administered questionnaires provide better responses to sensitive behaviors compared to the more expensive face-to-face interviews, (2) given the natural clusters of universities and classes, sampling designs are generally straightforward and cost-efficient, and (3) universities are generally willing to provide the necessary mailing lists to researchers. Of course, mail surveys are not without their difficulties. Mail surveys tend to (1) obtain lower response rates compared to other methods, (2) lack control over whether the intended respondent completed the questionnaire, (3) lack control over proper questionnaire skips and item non-response, and (4) require greater post survey data cleaning. In addition, regardless of the mode of administration, college surveys can be hampered by the quality of the sampling frames provided by universities, and, for multi-site surveys, multiple research ethics board approvals are a growing requirement.

More recently, given the high internet coverage of college students, web-based survey methods are becoming more frequently employed (Pealer and Weiler, 2003) and evaluated (McCabe et al., 2002). The strengths of web-based methods for college students include (1) reduced costs, (2) shorter data collection periods, (3) automatic data entry, and (4) excellent population coverage. On the other hand, the weaknesses include (1) perceived security issues, (2) sample frame access—not all universities allow distribution or access to their email lists, (3) a sizeable percentage of students do not regularly use their university affiliated URL, and (4) higher non-response rates.

Several evaluations have suggested that web methods are feasible, especially for the college population that has full access to the internet (Couper, 2000; Pealer and Weiler, 2003). The dominant concern regarding the web methodology is the potential bias caused by lower response rates of web surveys compared to mail surveys (Couper, 2000), although some studies have found the opposite (McCabe et al., 2002).

More critical to our concern is the nature of mode differences for alcohol and other drug use. Again, the evidence remains somewhat mixed. Although there is a notable mode difference showing higher reports of drug use for self-administered versus computer-assisted methods (Wright et al., 1998), such a difference seems to be less pervasive in the college population. Indeed, several studies have noted minimal drug use differences between web and mail methods (Bongers et al., 1998; Miller et al., 2002). The most notable of these studies is based on a survey of

7,000 undergraduates attending a large Midwestern university in 2001 (McCabe et al., 2002). Students were randomly assigned to either the web or mail mode. The results showed that, compared to the mail mode, the web sample more closely matched the target population and also had a higher response rate. Moreover, after controlling for design differences, there were no significant mode differences in data quality or in rates of alcohol and other drug use.

In sum, the use of web-based methods comes with its own unique set of difficulties for substance use researchers, but it is likely that such methods will become more commonly employed and developed and improved.

4.   HIGH RISK AND HIDDEN POPULATION SURVEYS

We have noted that a serious limitation of general population surveys is that the "hard-to-reach", "hidden" and "high-risk" populations are often excluded either by design, such as being excluded from the target population (e.g., students not enrolled in school, individuals without a permanent home), by respondent loss (e.g., absent students, non-participating respondents), or by the unreported drug use of respondents. In the drug use field this includes populations such as the homeless, street youth, prison detainees, HIV positive individuals and even mainstream drug-using populations (e.g., white-collar executives). Indeed, the stigmatization of some drug-using populations makes them difficult to list, locate and interview when approached by unknown researchers (Lambert, 1990).

Consequently, in order to gain access to such populations, it is often necessary to employ non-probability methods such as convenience or judgment samples. Indeed, such studies have made important contributions to the drug use field historically (Becker, 1953; Goode, 1970; Lindesmith, 1947), and more currently as well (Biernacki, 1986; Murphy et al., 1989; Williams, 1989; Zinberg, 1984).

Clearly, the major weakness of non probability based convenience samples is their inability to generalize to the population. Yet, although there have been technical means to draw probability samples from hidden populations (e.g., Goodman, 1961; Sudman et al., 1988), there are several reasons for the use of convenience samples (Faugier and Sargeant, 1997). Indeed, many contend that traditional random sampling methods are not viable for many drug-using populations (Griffiths et al., 1993; Hendricks and Blanken, 1992; Wiebel, 1990).

Methodologically, random surveys generally miss the hidden groups that typically have higher rates of drug use, and the standardized interview methods are not conducive to the flexibility and extensiveness of data collection typically conducted in convenience samples. Practically, random surveys require extensive resources. As well, they do not have the same capacity as convenience methods to encourage drug users to cooperate (Griffiths et al., 1993), and it is difficult to accumulate large numbers of deviant drug users.

In the drug use field, non-random samples include a wide array of strategies, the most common of which have been link-tracing studies, such as snowball sampling (Adler, 1990; Biernacki, 1986; French, 1993; Inciardi, 1993), and respondent-driven sampling (Heckathorn, 1997), and privileged access interviews (Griffiths et al., 1993). It is comforting to some that comparisons between convenience and representative samples have found many similarities (Erickson et al., 1994; Topp et al., 2004); yet, we must recognize that the absence of randomization means that we cannot be sure to what extent samples differ with respect to unmeasured variables.

A more critical issue to be considered by researchers is whether the substantive nature of the study requires generalization to the population, and hence a random sample. If the research objective is to study local social processes related to drug use, there is no need for a random sample. Indeed, there is a growing movement that probability and non-probability methods be viewed as complementary since the weaknesses of one are the strengths of the other (Faugier and Sargeant, 1997).

5. NEEDS AND CHALLENGES

The current state of data collection methods used in drug-use surveys has been discussed above. The needs and challenges facing drug use researchers require additional attention. More work needs to be done in developing and validating drug-use harm screeners similar to the Alcohol Use Disorders Identification Test (AUDIT) (Babor et al., 2001). Many of the large-scale surveys incorporate DSM (American Psychological Association, 1994) symptoms and perhaps diagnoses, but many drug users experience drug-related harms, and cause harms to others, that are not captured by DSM criteria. Moreover, it is important to assess the magnitude of harm before it develops into a clinical disorder. Fortunately, there is some work developing in this area (Adamson and Sellman, 2003), one example of which is a screener being developed by the World Health Organization (WHO ASSIST Working Group, 2002).

We need more research assessing trends in the relationship between the self-reporting of drug use and societal stigma. We tend to hold the assumption that, although our estimates of drug use are downwardly biased, that our estimates of trends over time are unbiased—which should be the case if the level of under-reporting remains constant. Yet, there is little empirical work to substantiate this assumption and the impact of changes of public perceptions about drug use.

There are also perennial challenges facing drug use researchers. The key challenge is to maintain, and where possible increase, response rates. Although we know that non-respondents often differ from respondents, we still lack a complete understanding regarding their impact on drug-use estimates, and to what extent we could employ such knowledge to increase participation.

REFERENCES

Abdullah, A.S., Fielding, R., and Hedley, A.J. (2002). Patterns of cigarette smoking, alcohol use and other substance use among Chinese university students in Hong Kong. *American Journal of Addiction* 11(3), pp. 235–246.

Adamson, S. and Sellman, J. (2003). A prototype screening instrument for cannabis use disorder: The Cannabis Use Disorders Identification Test (CUDIT) in an alcohol-dependent clinical sample. *Drug and Alcohol Review*, 22(3), pp. 309–315.

Adlaf, E.M., Gliksman, L., Demers, A., and Newton-Taylor, B. (2003). Illicit drug use among Canadian university undergraduates. *Canadian Journal of Nursing Research*, 35(1), pp. 24–43.

Adlaf, E.M., and Paglia, A. (2003). Drug Use Among Ontario Students: Detailed OSDUS Findings, 1977–2001: Centre for Addiction and Mental Health, Toronto.

Adler, P. (1990). Ethnographic research on hidden populations: Penetrating the Drug World. In: E. Lambert (Ed.), *The Collection and Interpretation of Data from Hidden Populations. NIDA Monograph 98*. National Institute on Drug Abuse, Rockville, MD.

American Psychological Association. (1994). *Diagnostic and Statistical Manual of Mental Disorders*, 4th Edition, American Psychological Association, Washington, D.C.

Anderman, C., Cheadle, A., Curry, S., Diehr, P., Shultz, L., and Wagner, E. (1995). Selection bias related to parental consent in school-based research. *Evaluation Review*, 19, pp. 663–674.

Aquilino, W.S. (1992). Telephone versus face-to-face interviewing for household drug use surveys. *International Journal of Addictions*, 27, pp. 71–91.

Aquilino, W.S. (1994). Interview mode effects in surveys of drug and alcohol use: A field experiment. *Public Opinion Quarterly*, 58, pp. 210–240.

Babor, T.R., Higgins-Biddle, J.C., Saunders, J.B., and Monteiro, M.G. (2001). *The Alcohol Use Disorders Identification Test: Guidelines for Use in Primary Care*. World Health Organization, Geneva.

Becker, H.S. (1953). Becoming a marijuana user. *American Journal of Sociology*, 54, pp. 235–242.

Bell, R., Wechsler, H., and Johnston, L.D. (1997). Correlates of college student marijuana use: Results of a US National Survey. *Addiction*, 92(5), pp. 571–581.

Biernacki, P. (1986). *Pathways from Heroin Addiction*. Temple University Press, Philadelphia.

Bongers, I.M.B. and van Oers, J.A.M. (1998). Mode effects on self-reported alcohol use and problem drinking: Mail questionnaires and personal interviewing compared. *Journal of Studies on Alcohol*, 59, pp. 280–285.

Brener, N., Billy, J., and Grady, W. (2003). Assessment of factors affecting the validity of self-reported health-risk behavior among adolescents: Evidence from the scientific literature. *Journal of Adolescent Health*, 33(6), pp. 436–457.

Centers for Disease Control and Prevention 2004. About the BRFSS (October 2004); http://www.cdc.gov/brfss/about.htm.

Couper, M.P. (2000). Web surveys: A review of issues and approaches. *Public Opinion Quarterly*, 64, pp. 464–494.

de Leeuw, E.D., and van der Zouwen, J. (1988). Data quality in telephone and face-to-face surveys: A comparative meta-analysis. In: R. M. Groves, P. Biemer, L. Lyberg, J. L. Massey, W. Nicholls II, and J. Waksberg (Eds.), *Telephone Survey Methodology*. Wiley, New York.

Dent, C.W., Galaif, J., Sussman, S., Stacy, A., Burton, D., and Flay, B.R. (1993). Demographic, psychosocial and behavioral differences in samples of actively and passively consented adolescents. *Addictive Behaviors*, 18, pp. 51–56.

Dent, C.W., Sussman, S., and Stacy, A. (1997). The impact of a written parental consent policy on estimates from a school-based drug use survey. *Evaluation Review*, 21, pp. 698–712.

Erickson, P., Adlaf, E.M., Smart, R.G., and Murray, G.F. (1994). *The Steel Drug: Cocaine and Crack in Perspective*. Lexington Books, New York.

Faugier, J. and Sargeant, M. (1997). Sampling hard to reach populations. *Journal of Advanced Nursing*, 26, pp. 790–797.

French, J. (1993). Pipe dreams: Crack and the life in Philadelphia and Newark. In: M. Ratner (Ed.), *Crack Pipe as Pimp*. Lexington Books, New York.

Gfroerer, J. (1985). Influences of Privacy on Self-Reported Drug Use by Youths. In: B.A. Rouse, N.J. Kozel, and L. G. Richards (Eds.), *Self-Report Methods of Estimating Drug Use. NIDA Research Monograph 57*. Department of Health and Human Services, Rockville.

Gfroerer, J. and Hughes, A.L. (1992). Collecting data on illicit drug use by phone. In: C.F. Turner, J.T. Lessler, and J.C. Gfroerer (Eds.), *Survey Measurement of Drug Use: Methodological Studies*. Department of Health and Human Services, Washington, D.C.

Gfroerer, J., Wright, D., and Kopstein, A. (1997). Prevalence of youth substance use: the impact of methodological differences between two national surveys. *Drug and Alcohol Dependence*, 47, pp. 19–30.

Gfroerer, J.C., and Hughes, A.L. (1991). The feasibility of collecting drug abuse data by telephone. *Public Health Rep*, 106(4), pp. 384–393.

Gliksman, L., Demers, A., Adlaf, E.M., Newton-Taylor, B., and Schmidt, K. (2000). Canadian Campus Survey 1998. Centre for Addiction and Mental Health, Toronto.

Goode, E. (1970). *The Marihuana Smokers*. Basic Books, New York.

Goodman, L. (1961). Snowball sampling. *Annals of Mathematical Statistics*, 32, pp. 245–268.

Gribble, J., Miller, H., Catania, J., Pollack, L., and Turner, C.F. (2000). The impact of T-ACASI interviewing on reported drug use among men who have sex with men. *Substance Use and Misuse*, pp. 869–890.

Griffiths, P., Gossop, M., Powis, B., and Strang, J. (1993). Reaching hidden populations of drug users by privileged access interviews: methodological and practical issues. *Addiction*, 88, pp. 1617–1626.

Griffiths, P., and McKetin, R. (2003). Developing a global perspective on drug consumption patterns and trends—the challenge for drug epidemiology. *Bulletin on Narcotics*, LV(1 and 2), pp. 1–8.

Groves, R.M., Fowler, F.J., Couper, M.P., Lepkowski, J.M., Singer, E., and Tourangeau, R. (2004). *Survey Methodology*. Wiley, New York.

Grulich, A., de Visser, R., Smith, A., Rissel, C., and Richters, J. (2003). Sex in Australia: injecting and sexual risk behaviour in a representative sample of adults. *Australian and New Zealand Journal of Public Health*, 27(2), pp. 242–250.

Guttmacher, S., Weitzman, B.C., Kapadia, F., and Weinberg, S.L. (2002). Classroom-based surveys of adolescent risk-taking behaviors: Reducing the bias of absenteeism. *Amercian Journal of Public Health*, 92(2), pp. 235–237.

Hall, W., Carless, J., Homel, P., Flaherty, B., and Reilly, C. (1991). The characteristics of cocaine users among young adults in Sydney. *Medical Journal of Australia*, 155, pp. 11–14.

Hallfors, D. and Iritani, B. (2002). Local and state school-based substance use surveys. *Evaluation Review*, 25(4), pp. 418–437.

Harrington, K., Binkley, D., Reynolds, K., Duvall, R., Copeland, J., Franklin, F., and Raczynski, J. (1997). Recruitment issues in school-based research: Lessons learned from the High 5 Alabama Project. *Journal of School Health*, 67, pp. 415–421.

Heckathorn, D. (1997). Respondent-driven sampling: A new approach to the study of hidden populations. *Social Problems*, 44, pp. 174–199.

Hendricks, V. and Blanken, P. (1992). Snowball sampling: Theoretical and practical considerations. In V. Hendricks and P. Blanken (Eds.), *Snowball Sampling: A Pilot Study on Cocaine Use*. IVO, Rotterdam.

Henry, K.L., Smith, E.A., and Hopkins, A. (2002). The effect of active parental consent on the ability to generalize the results of an alcohol, tobacco, and other drug prevention trial to rural adolescents. *Evaluation Review*, 26(6), pp. 645–655.

Hibell, B., Andersson, B., Ahlstrom, S., Balakireva, O., Bjarnason, T., Kokkevi, A., and Morgan, M. (2000). *The 1999 ESPAD Report: Alcohol and Other Drug Use Among Students in 30 European Countries*. Stockholm: The Swedish Council for Information on Alcohol and Other Drugs; The Pompidou Group at the Council of Europe.

Inciardi, J. (1993). Kingrats, chicken heads, slow necks, freaks and blood suckers: A glimpse at the Miami sex-for-crack market. In: M. Ratner (Ed.), *Crack Pipe as Pimp*. Lexington, New York.

Johnson, T.P. and Mott, J.A. (2001). The reliability of self-reported age of onset of tobacco, alcohol and illicit drug use. *Addiction*, 96, pp. 1187–1198.

Johnston, L.D. and O'Malley, P.M. (1985). Issues of validity and population coverage in student surveys of drug use. In: B. A. Rouse, N. J. Kozel, and L. G. Richards (Eds.), *Self-Report Methods Of Estimating Drug Use: Meeting Current Challenges to Validity*. Department of Health and Human Services, Washington, D.C.

Johnston, L.D., O'Malley, P.M., and Bachman, J.G. (2002). *Monitoring the Future National Survey Results on Drug Use, 1975–2001. Volume I: Secondary School Students*. National Institute on Drug Abuse, Bethesda, MD.

Johnston, L.D., O'Malley, P.M., Bachman, J.G., and Schulenberg, J.E. (2004). *Monitoring the Future National Survey Results on Drug Use, 1975–2003. Volume I: Secondary School Students*. National Institute on Drug Abuse, Bethesda, MD.

Kerber, L., and Wallisch, L. (1999). *1997 Texas Survey of Substance Use Among University Students*. Texas Commission on Alcohol and Drug Abuse. Austin, Texas.

Kilpatrick, D., Ruggiero, K., Acierno, R., Saunders, B., Resnick, H., and Best, C. (2003). Violence and risk of PTSD. major depression, substance abuse/dependence, and comorbidity: Results from the National Survey of Adolescents. *Journal of Consulting and Clinical Psychology*, 71(4), pp. 692–700.

Lambert, E. (1990). *The Collection and Interpretation of Data from Hidden Populations. NIDA Monograph 98*. National Institute on Drug Abuse, Rockville.

Lindesmith, R. (1947). *Opiate Addiction*. Principa Press, Bloomington.

MacNeil, P. and Webster, I. (1997). Canada's Alcohol and Other Drugs Survey 1994: A Discussion of the Findings, *Canada's Alcohol and Other Drugs Survey 1994: A Discussion of the Findings*. Minister of Public Works and Government and Services Canada, Ottawa.

Mangione, T., Hingson, R., and Barrett, J. (1982). Collecting sensitive data: A comparison of three survey strategies. *Sociological Methods and Research*, 10, pp. 337–346.

Mangweth, B., Pope, H.G., Ionescu-Pioggia, M., Kinzl, J., and Biebl, W. (1997). Drug use and lifestyle among college students in Austria and the United States. *Substance Use and Misuse*, 32(4), pp. 461–473.

Martinez, J.M., Carmen Del Rio, M.d., Lopez, N., and Alvarez, F.J. (1999). Illegal drug-using trends among students in a Spanish University in the last decade (1984–1994). *Substance Use and Misuse*, 34(9), pp. 1281–1297.

McCabe, S.E., Boyd, C.J., Couper, M.P., Crawford, S., and D'Arcy, H. (2002). Mode effects for collecting alcohol and other drug use data: Web and U.S. mail. *Journal of Studies on Alcohol*, 63, pp. 755–761.

Medina-Mora, M.E., Castro, S., Campillo-Serrano, C., and Gomez-Mont, F. (1981). Validity and reliability of a high school drug use questionnaire among Mexican students. *Bulletin on Narcotics*, 33(4), pp. 67–76.

Meilman, P., Gaylor, M., Turco, J., and Stone, J. (1990). Drug use among college undergraduates: Current use and 10 year trends. *International Journal of the Addictions*, 25, pp. 1025–1036.

Midanik, L. and Greenfield, T. (2003). Telephone versus in-person interviews for alcohol use: Results of the 2000 National Alcohol Survey. *Drug and Alcohol Dependence*, 72(3), pp. 209–214.

Miller, E.T., Neal, D.J., Roberts, L.J., Baer, J.S., Cressler, S.O., Metrik, J., and Marlatt, A.T. (2002). Test-retest reliability of alcohol measures: Is there a difference between internet-based assessment and traditional methods? *Psychology of Addictive Behaviors*, 16(1), pp. 56–63.

Mohler-Kuo, M., Lee, J., and Wechsler, H. (2003). Trends in marijuana and other illicit drug use among college students: Results from the 4 Harvard School of Public Health College Alcohol Study Surveys: 1993–2001. *Journal of American College Health*, 52(1), pp. 17–24.

Murphy, S.B., Reinarman, C., and Waldorf, D. (1989). An 11-year follow-up of a network of cocaine users. *British Journal of Addictions*, 84, pp. 427–436.

O'Donnell, L., Duran, R., San Doval, A., Breslin, M., Juhn, G., and Stueve, A. (1997). Obtaining written parent permission for school-based health surveys of urban young adolescents. *Journal of Adolescent Health*, 21(6), pp. 376–383.

O'Malley, P.M. and Johnston, L.D. (2002). Epidemiology of Alcohol and Other Drug Use among American College Students. *Journal of Studies on Alcohol, Supplement No. 14*, pp. 23–39.

O'Malley, P.M., Johnston, L.D., Bachman, J.G., and Schulenberg, J. (2000). Comparison of confidential versus anonymous survey procedures: Effects on reporting of drug use and related attitudes and beliefs in a national study of students. *Journal of Drug Issues*, 30(1), pp. 35–54.

Pealer, L. and Weiler, R. (2003). Guidelines for designing a web-delivered college health risk behavior survey: Lessons learned from the University of Florida Health Behavior Survey. *Health Promotion Practice*, 4(2), pp. 171–179.

Pope, H.G., Jr., Ionescu-Pioggia, M., and Pope, K.W. (2001). Drug use and life style among college undergraduates: a 30-year longitudinal study. *Am J Psychiatry*, 158(9), pp. 1519–1521.

Prendergast, M.L. (1994). Substance use and abuse among college students: A review of recent literature. *Journal of American College Health*, 43(3), pp. 99–113.

Rootman, I. and Smart, R.G. (1985). A comparison of alcohol, tobacco and drug use as determined from household and school surveys. *Drug and Alcohol Dependence*, 16, pp. 89–94.

Schober, S., Caces, M., Pergamit, M., and Branden, L. (1992). Effects of mode of administration on reporting of drug use in the National Longitudinal Survey. In: C.F. Turner, J.T. Lessler, and J. Gfroerer (Eds.), *Survey Measurement of Drug Use: Methodological Studies*. National Institute on Drug Abuse, Rockville, MD.

Severson, H. and Ary, D.V. (1983). Sampling bias due to consent procedures with adolescents. *Addictive Behaviors*, 8, pp. 433–437.

Smart, R.G., Hughes, P.H., Johnston, L.D., Anumonye, A., Khant, U., Medina Mora, M.E., Navaratnam, V., Poshyachinda, V., Varma, V.K., and Wadud, K.A. (1980). A Methodology for Student Drug-Use Surveys. World Health Organization, Geneva.

Smart, R.G. and Ogborne, A.C. (2000). Drug use and drinking among students in 36 countries. *Addictive Behaviors*, 25(3), pp. 455–460.

Strote, J., Lee, J.E., and Wechsler, H. (2002). Increasing MDMA use among college students: results of a national survey. *Journal of Adolescent Health*, 30(1), pp. 64–72.

Substance Abuse and Mental Health Services Administration (2004). Results from the 2003 National Survey on Drug Use and Health: National Findings, SAMHSA, Rockville, MD.

Sudman, S. (2001). Examining substance abuse data collection methodologies. *Journal of Drug Issues*, 31(3), pp. 695–716.

Sudman, S., Sirken, M.G., and Cowan, C. (1988). Sampling rare and elusive populations. *Science*, 240, pp. 991–996.

Sykes, W., and Collins, M. (1988). Effects of mode of interview: Experiments in the UK. In R.M. Groves, P. Biemer, L. Lyberg, J.L. Massey, W. Nicholls II, and J. Waksberg (Eds.), *Telephone Survey Methodology*. Wiley, New York.

Topp, L., Barker, B., and Degenhardt, L. (2004). The external validity of results derived from ecstasy users recruited using purposive sample strategies. *Drug and Alcohol Dependence*, 73, pp. 33–40.

Turner, C.F., Lessler, J.T., and Devore, J. (1992). Effects of mode of administration and wording on reporting of drug use. In: C.F. Turner, J.T. Lessler, and J. Gfroerer (Eds.), *Survey Measurement of Drug Use: Methodological Studies*. National Institute on Drug Abuse, Rockville.

Turner, C.F., Lessler, J.T., and Gfroerer, J.C. (1992). Survey Measurement of Drug Use: Methodological Studies, *Survey Measurement of Drug Use: Methodological Studies*. Department of Health and Human Services, Washington, D.C.

Turner, C.F., Miller, H., Smith, T., Cooley, P., and Rogers, S. (1996). Telephone audio computer-assisted self-interviewing (T-ACASI) and survey measurements of sensitive behaviors: Preliminary results. In R. Banks, J. Fairgrieve, and L. Gerrard (Eds.), *Survey and Statistical Computing 1996*. Association for Survey Computing, Chesham, UK.

United Nations Office on Drugs and Crime (2003). *Conducting School Surveys on Drug Abuse: Global Assessment Programme on Drug Abuse: Toolkit Module 3*. United Nations, New York.

Wallisch, L.D. (2001). *2000 Texas Survey of Substance Use Among Adults*. Texas Commission on Alcohol and Drug Abuse. Austin, Texas.

Webb, E.A., Ashtoa, C.H., Kelly, P. and Kamali, F. (1996). Alcohol and drug use in UK university students. *Lancet*, 348(9032), pp. 922–925.

White, V.M., Hill, D.J., and Effendi, Y. (2004). How does active parental consent influence the findings of drug-use surveys in schools? *Evaluation Review*, 28(3), pp. 246–260.

WHO ASSIST Working Group (2002). Alcohol, smoking and substance involvement screening test (ASSIST): Development, reliability and feasibility. *Addiction*, 97(9), pp. 1183–1194.

Wiebel, W. (1990). Identifying and gaining access to hidden populations. In: E. Lambert (Ed.), *The Collection and Interpretation of Data from Hidden Populations. NIDA Monograph 98*. National Institute on Drug Abuse, Rockville, MD.

Wilkins, C., Bhatta, K., Pledger, M., and Casswell, S. (2003). Ecstasy use in New Zealand: findings from the 1998 and 2001 National Drug Surveys. *New Zealand Medical Journal*, 116, U383.

Williams, T. (1989). *The Cocaine Kids: The Inside Story of a Teenage Drug Ring*. Addison-Wesley Publishing, New York.

Wright, D.L., Aquilino, W.S., and Supple, A. (1998). A comparison of computer-assisted and paper-and-pencil self-administered questionnaires in a survey of smoking, alcohol and other drug use. *Public Opinion Quarterly*, 62, pp. 331–353.

Zinberg, N.E. (1984). *Drug, Set and Setting: The Basis for Controlled Intoxicant Use*. Yale University Press, New Haven.

8

Indirect Methods to Estimate Prevalence

Matthew Hickman and Colin Taylor

MATTHEW HICKMAN • Imperial College
COLIN TAYLOR • European Monitoring Centre for Drugs and Drug Addiction

1. OVERVIEW

The first point to be made is that there are very good reasons to estimate the prevalence of problem drug use—which in this chapter refers almost exclusively to injecting drug use, heroin/opiate, and crack-cocaine use. The second is that population or general household surveys, which usually represent the best direct method of prevalence estimation, are not the answer for estimating these forms of problem drug use. Injecting drug users and opiate/ crack-cocaine users are comparatively rare and a largely "hidden" population—that is, they are hard to access by the usual means and are not readily accessed through surveys or administrative records. Counting the number of problem drug users in contact with treatment, police or other services is not sufficient as a prevalence estimate, since only a proportion of the target population is in contact with these services at any time and there is no available base or denominator.

Indirect methods offer an alternative way of estimating prevalence; some of these have been borrowed from animal ecology and some also are in use for other public health problems. In general indirect methods utilize routinely collected data sources. The discussion below presents examples of their use for estimating the prevalence of injecting drug use. The key to improving the evidence on the prevalence of problem drug use centers on improving the routine collection and integration of data on problem drug users that have as a goal "prevalence estimation".

1.1. Why Estimate Prevalence?

There is a growing recognition that policy-makers require evidence on the national and local prevalence of the problem. Gone are the days when, in response to one of the earliest attempts to estimate the prevalence of heroin use in the United States, a reviewer commented, "why bother estimating incidence and prevalence— would policy be any different if [there were] 300,000 or 3 million". (Hunt, 1974; Rittenhouse et al. 1997). Though some doubt whether policy is sufficiently evidence based, the growth in manuals on how to estimate prevalence and examples of prevalence estimates in support of policy is testament to the interest and importance of providing good evidence on prevalence (See, for example, Hser et al., 1992; GAP, 2002; EMCDDA, 1997, 2000; Hickman et al., 2003; Maxwell, 2000).

Prevalence estimates are required primarily in three key areas, service planning and resource allocation, monitoring key targets, and public health surveillance/epidemiology.

1.1.1.   Service Planning and Resource Allocation

The prevalence of a disease can be central to arguments for securing resources for an appropriate response in terms of treatment and other measures to reduce the associated harm. While it is the consequent public health and social problems associated with drug use that are directly or indirectly addressed, it is the overall level of prevalence that is frequently highlighted as a summary measure of these problems.

1.1.2.   Monitoring Key Targets

The prevalence of problem drug use is often a component of local or national measures of the "coverage" of treatment or harm reduction. For example, in the United Kingdom the government is monitoring the proportion of problem drug users in contact with treatment. Globally, countries have been asked to estimate and monitor the proportion of injecting drug users in contact with services that seek to prevent Human Immunodeficiency Virus (HIV) infection.

1.1.3.   Public Health Surveillance/Epidemiology

Prevalence estimates assist the interpretation and measurement of harms associated with drug use. The burden of HIV, Hepatitis C Virus, fatal overdose, and drug related crime associated with drug use in the population as a whole is related both to the level of risk behaviors found among problem drug users and to the prevalence of problem drug use itself. For example, the attributable risk fraction of mortality that may be caused by injecting/opiate use on adult mortality can be estimated by combining information on the prevalence of injecting/opiate use in the population and the Standardized Mortality Ratio of drug related mortality compared to the general population. (Bargagli et al., forthcoming)

Traditionally, the prevalence of an important public health problem would be one of the outputs of a public health surveillance system. The most common modern definition of "public health surveillance" is "the ongoing systematic collection, analysis, and interpretation of data on specific health events for use in the planning, implementation, and evaluation of public health programs" (CDC, 1988); often paraphrased as "information for action". (CDC, 1992). Public health surveillance systems for many infectious diseases are well established, and in developing countries have been extended to chronic diseases. Drug addiction was mentioned as a likely candidate for surveillance in 1968 (Berkelman and Buehler, 1991) though little work has been done to outline what a surveillance system for "drug addiction" would entail. We will come back to the principles of public health surveillance in the concluding section.

1.2.   Why Indirect and Not Direct?

Direct methods for estimating levels of any behavior in a population (e.g. population or household surveys) are often considered a 'gold standard' for measuring prevalence, and they can be very effective in monitoring common drug using behaviors such as tobacco or alcohol. However, direct methods are inefficient and ineffective when measuring the prevalence of rare, more covert, more stigmatized and more problematic forms of drug use, such as injecting or heroin or crack-cocaine use (NRC, 2001). Therefore there are multiple opportunities for bias. For instance, injecting drug users (IDU) or crack-cocaine users are less likely than non-problematic drug users to live in households included in general household surveys; IDU/crack users may be less likely to participate in the survey even if asked; and injection or crack use may be less likely to be reported than other forms of drug use.

Two studies illustrate these points. First, an analysis of combined surveys of over 90,000 subjects in the United States which presented cases by year of initiation failed to detect any change in the incidence of heroin use between 1960 and 1990—which is highly unlikely to be an accurate picture of use over that time period. (Gfroerer and Brodsky, 1992). Second, the 2001 British Crime Survey, with a sample size of over 30,000 found less than 50 people reporting that they used heroin in the last month, giving an estimate for Britain of 33,000, which is implausible as it falls short of the number of heroin users presenting to treatment sites (Aust et al., 2002).

Equally ineffective is an alternative strategy of compiling a register of known injecting drug users or crack-cocaine users. This is a common response in the monitoring of several diseases such as cancers, AIDS, Congenital Heart Defect, other congenital disorders, and childhood diabetes, but such an approach even if it combined multiple data sources would substantially under-estimate the prevalence of problem drug use. In theory, it is possible to ascertain a complete reporting of *all* diagnosed cases of diabetes or AIDS. However, in any one year a substantial proportion of problem drug users will not be in contact with *any* service so that a contact report could be made. In fact, it is not known what proportion of users over their injecting life-course will *not* have any contact with services.

2. INDIRECT ESTIMATION METHODS

The rationale for indirect estimation methods is that direct methods are impracticable or unreliable, and a simple count of known cases or instances will not suffice. In the absence of a ready-made sampling frame that covers problem drug users (PDU), the classical starting-point for direct methods, investigators turn to other means (Suzman et al., 1988). Animal ecologists face the same problem wanting to know the number or abundance of a specific animal in an area. As a result a number of indirect methods, appropriate to different animals and habitats, have been developed in ecology (Seber, 1982). The parallels between animal ecologists and epidemiologists (both estimating "elusive" and "hidden" populations) seems ready-made for injecting drug use and often have been noted, especially given

Table 1. Potential Data Sources for Indirect Estimation Methods

Data Source	Example
Specialist drug treatment	Drug users on methadone, attending treatment agencies, or in residential care
Low threshold drug agencies	Drug users attending drop-in sites or contacted by out-reach workers
Needle exchange	Drug users registered at needle exchange program (SEP)
Casualty	Drug users attending casualty because of an overdose or other problem
Laboratory	Drug users tested for HIV, HCV or HBV
Police/Prison	Drug users arrested or imprisoned for drug offences, Drug users arrested or imprisoned for other crimes but screened for drug problems
Probation	Drug users on probation
Social services—assessments	Drug users assessed by local social services
Hostels for drug users	Drug users living in hostels
Addict Registers	Drug users reported to a central register
Overdose deaths	Number of deaths due to opiate overdose

the widespread use of capture-recapture methods. However, we caution against reading too much into the parallel, since normally the conduct of the studies and the statistical models are very different.

The starting point for indirect estimation is having data on a sample of problem drug users (referred to as the observed data set), which though may be partial provides some information on the characteristics and number of problem drug users. The aim of the indirect estimation methods is to analyze the observed data set or combine it with other information to estimate the "proportion of the [problem drug use] target population sampled within the observed data set", and thereby to arrive at an estimate of the prevalence. Table 1 shows some potential data sources used in prevalence estimation, some of which may be available locally or could be generated.

Indirect methods use these data sources as their raw material and seek to estimate the sampling intensity, i.e. the proportion of the total number of problem drug users sampled in the study. Often this requires having sufficient information on the data sources to match against subjects who appear on two or more data sources; or to obtain other information on how a specific data source (in Table 1) relates to the overall population of problem drug users. The question of this approach then is whether multiple data sources or samples can be used to ascertain the proportion of subjects observed or not observed at a particular source. In this problem of 'incomplete ascertainment' over multiple data sources, it is important to explicitly recognize that many subjects (problem drug users) are unknown to any one or all of the data sources. The disadvantage of indirect methods is that a series of assumptions are made regarding the relationship of the observed data set(s) to the numbers of problem drug users in the target population (these are summarized below). Furthermore, violation of the assumptions may lead to bias so that the precision of the estimates or how accurately the model represents the target population cannot be empirically tested. Table 2 summarizes a number of indirect estimation methods.

Therefore the central problem in designing indirect estimation studies is obtaining a random sample of problem drug users in first instance. While it is relatively easy in direct estimation methods to check that a sample has been drawn from the sampling frame in a random manner, at least in so far as the design has been properly operationalized, it is far more difficult to make a similar assessment when using indirect methods. A range of assumptions is required that in essence ensure two things: firstly, that the sample behaves, in statistical terms, as though drawn from a conceptual (but unattainable) sampling frame; and secondly, that the required design procedures are operationally valid (i.e., correctly identifies the sample and its relationship with the total population).

These assumptions (some or all of which apply to the various indirect methods) include the following: having a stable population, having equal probabilities that a single subject will be observed in a given data source, matching of subject characteristics can be made across data sources, and that appearing on a data source is independent of appearing on others.

1. Stability of Population: The number of drug users entering or exiting from the population over the period of study is negligible in practical terms. Technically, if the 'time spent at risk of being observed' is known, then corrections can be made to allow for a shifting population—but in practice, this is never the case.

2. Equi-probable sampling: There is an equal probability of any subject being observed at a given data source. Technically, where multiple data sources are used, this requirement need apply only to one of the sources.

3. Matching definitions: Definitions of groups of subjects and the identification of individual subjects should match correctly across data sources. Technically, this implies no misclassification of subjects as IDU or PDU, or false negative or positive matches of subjects between data sources.

4. Source conditional independence: If a subject appears on one data source he/she is not more or less likely to appear on another data source, i.e., positive or negative dependence. Technically, in ecology studies it refers to trap fascination or trap avoidance, or significant interactions in statistical parlance. In theory dependence can be adjusted for in the analysis, except if in a study of n data sources where there are n-way interactions. For example, with two samples the data sources must be independent, with three data sources there must be no 3-way interaction and so on.

In practice, all the methods presume that the data sources are broadly representative of the population being studied, or at least aim for that as the safest design. It has been noted (Cormack,1992) that in contrast to direct estimation there

Table 2. Indirect Methods of Estimating Prevalence of Injection/Problem Drug
Use (IDU/PDU)

Method	Summary	Example
Multiplier methods	Combines data on number of known IDU (benchmark, eg, number in treatment, tested for HIV, fatal OD) and information on proportion of IDU that would appear on benchmark (multiplier, e.g proportion in treatment, tested for HIV, died of fatal OD) to estimate total IDU population.	See Archibald (2001), Hartnoll (1985)
Capture-recapture methods	Takes and matches 3 or more data sources of IDU (eg. Treatment, arrest, syringe exchange), analyses the overlap between the data sources using log-linear models to estimate the number of IDU "unobserved" by the data sets and the total number of IDU	See Hook and Regal (1995), Hickman (2004)
Capture-recapture methods—open populations	Analyses repeat captures/surveys over time (e.g. number of occasions sex workers observed over time, or re-attendances by IDU at injecting room) to estimate total population size and its rate of change over time	See McGeganey (1992)
Truncated Poisson	Takes single data source (e.g. attendances at treatment, arrests, visitis to SEP) and analyses frequency of 1, 2, etc attendances in order to probability of attending once, twice etcc and predict probability and proportion of subjects attending 0 times, and estimate total IDU population.	See Hay (2003)
Enhanced/event Based multipliers	Collects data on event history from multiple data sources/benchmarks (e.g. history of imprisonment, treatment, hostel use), combines them in order to adjust for biases, and combines them with benchmarks to estimate total number of IDU/PDU	See Simeone (1997)
Synthetic estimation	Takes estimates of IDU population in selected sites (usually generated by other indirect methods) and estimates number of IDU in other sites using proportional ratio or regression methods based on single or multiple indicators of IDU that are available in all areas (e.g. number of fatal OD, drug treatment and criminal justice data).	See Rhodes (1993), Frischer (2001)
Back-calculation	Uses information on trends in an observed end-point (e.g. fatal OD), combined with information on the incubation distribution (e.g. heroin/1DU cessation rate, OD and drug related mortality rate) to estimate incidence and prevalence of heroin/1DU use) over time.	See Law (2001), De Angelis (In press)

are no clear sample size calculations that can be made in advance of an analysis that could guarantee a level of reliability. Though as a general rule the greater the amount of data collected and the greater the sampling intensity the better (Wittes 1974). Furthermore, though some methods can generate confidence intervals using standard statistical equations, any uncertainty (or bias) arising from sampling the population is often far outweighed by uncertainty or bias arising from violation of the assumptions and uncertainty surrounding some of the data inputs. It is rarely possible to test empirically whether the final prevalence estimates are true. For this reason it is essential that the estimates are "evidence based" i.e. that the estimates are corroborated or consistent with other information, or other knowledge and expertise is used to help judge whether the estimates are credible. The methods generally used to make indirect prevalence estimates include: multiplier methods, capture-recapture, and others. The following sections discuss each of these methods, offering case studies as examples of their application.

2.1. Multiplier Methods

Multiplier methods (also referred to as ratio-estimation) were probably the first and most common methods for estimating the prevalence of problem drug use. Superficially versatile, easy to use and calculate, in theory they can use any of the data sources given in Table 1. Two elements are required: first, a data source usually called a "benchmark" (representing a known number of problem drug users that have experienced a particular event, such as treatment or arrest or overdose); second, an estimate of the proportion of all problem drug users that have been recorded in the benchmark (e.g. the proportion in treatment might be 1 in 10; or 1 in 50 arrested, or overdose mortality rate amongst problem users might be 1 in 100). The reciprocal of the proportion is termed the multiplier. The benchmark represents the known drug users and the proportion estimates the 'sampling intensity' that generated them. For example, if the benchmark were 3,000 and it was estimated that 20 percent of the population under investigation were recorded on the benchmark, the multiplier would be 5 (since 1/20percent = 5) and the estimated total would be calculated as 15,000 (that is, 5 * 3,000).

In essence, the multiplier is a two-source method (one source is the benchmark, the other is the data used to provide the estimate of the proportion and multiplier). The assumptions of the multiplier method are all those outlined above, i.e., the population of problem drug users needs to be stable and the same during the benchmark recording as during the multiplier estimation; the sample that is used to estimate the multiplier should be representative of the overall population of problem drug users, in practice not easily done; and, it is important that the definition used for the benchmark is precise and matches exactly that used in estimating the multiplier. As an example of this latter point, if arrest data are used for the benchmark then the multiplier needs to find the proportion of drug users arrested, not those charged or sentenced. Or again, if a number of treatment clinics' records over one year is the benchmark, then the multiplier must relate to attendance at those clinics over that year.

In the 1970s, mortality multipliers were used to estimate the prevalence of opiate use in the United States and United Kingdom (Andima et al., 1973; Hartnoll et al., 1985). For example, Hartnoll et al. (1985) multiplied the annual number of opiate overdose deaths by 50 to 100 on the basis that opiate overdose mortality rate was 1 percent to 2 percent per annum. Multiplier methods also have been applied to arrest data, treatment statistics and HIV reports (see box), and these methods continue to be used (Archibald et al., 2001; Frank et al., 1978; Parker et al., 1988; Godfrey et al., 2002; Dupont, 1973; Hall, 2000).

Various methods have been used to derive the multiplier, all attempting to approximate a random sample of drug users from which to estimate it. These include—not always successfully—site sampling methods (sampling drug users present at a representative set of geographical sites), and 'community sampling' (chain referral or snowball techniques that attempt to produce a representative sample of all drug users).

Nomination also has been used to obtain a multiplier (Parker et al., 1988). This describes a technique where a sample (e.g. injecting drug users) are asked questions about their friends or acquaintances (their nominees) that also are injecting drug users. For example, Parker and colleagues conducted a study with sixty IDU in the Wirral who were asked to nominate their five closest acquaintances and say how many were in treatment last year. The sixty IDU reported 300 other IDU. After removing duplicates this figure was reduced to 170 of whom 55 were identified as being in treatment giving a proportion of 32.4 percent and a multiplier of 3.1 (Parker et al., 1988).

Case Study 1 conducted by Archibald and colleagues (2001) for Toronto used as a benchmark laboratory reports of HIV test results that indicated injecting drug use as a risk factor and a survey of injectors from several Canadian cities asked

Case Study 1. Multiplier Study Based on HIV Tests in Toronto

Benchmark (B)	Number of HIV tests by injecting drug users in 1996—*Source: laboratory reports*	4050
Multiplier (M)	Proportion of injectors reporting getting an HIV test in the previous year—*Source: community recruited survey of injectors*	23% (multiplier = $1/0.23 = 4.35$)
Prevalence estimate	B * M (4050*4.35)	17,600

about being tested for HIV in the same year as the multiplier. In addition to showing how the multiplier method is applied, this example also illustrates the underlying problems with this approach:

- Is the benchmark complete and accurate? It may be necessary to adjust the benchmark, for example, to account for missing exposure information and/or HIV tests.
- Is the multiplier representative of the target population? This presents a greater problem. In this case study information from a community sample of IDUs recruited in a different year and city was used to derive the multiplier. Ideally, the multiplier should be obtained from a representative sample of problem drug users and collected over the time period and place corresponding to the benchmark data. In practice, however, random and representative samples of IDU are nigh on impractical to obtain.

Great caution needs to be exercised when using multiplier studies that are not confirmed, validated, or cross-checked with other information and other studies.

2.2. Capture Recapture

Capture-recapture methods were developed by animal ecologists to estimate animal abundance and the dynamics of animal populations (Begon, 1979). There are two principal types of model: closed and open population models. Open population models relax assumption #1(having a stable population) and because of the need for multiple independent data sets have had limited use in estimating the prevalence of problem drug use (see the two examples below). Closed population models with two data sources are more vulnerable to assumption #4 (having independent data sources) than those with three or more data sources, as it is not possible to test the independence of the two samples in the analysis.

Capture-recapture methods have been used extensively in epidemiology to adjust surveys, surveillance systems, and disease registers for under-ascertainment and therefore to estimate prevalence. (Chandra Sekar et al., 1949; Fienberg, 1992; Hook and Regal, 1995; International Working Group for Disease Monitoring and Forecasting, 1995). Bishop et al (1975) were the first to identify the potential for capture- recapture methods in estimating the prevalence of addiction, which since have been used in many cities worldwide (Hickman et al., 1999, 2004; Hay and McKegany, 1996; Squires et al., 1995; Hay, 2000; Brugha et al., 1998; Domingo-Salvaney et al., 1998, 1995; Bello and Chene, 1997; Kehoe et al., 1992; Comiskey and Barry, 2001; Duque-Portugal et al, 1994; Larson et al., 1994).

Ideally, capture-recapture involves the collection of three or more data sources of problem drug users with sufficient detail on the subjects to identify matches between data sources. Information on the number of matches between the data

Case Study 2a. Estimating Number of Injecting Drug Users in Bangkok, 1991

		Arrestees with urine positive for opiates (S2)		
		Yes	No	
Methadone	Yes	171	3893	4064
Maintenance	No	1369	?(x)	
(S1)				
		1540		N

So,

$$\text{population estimate, } N = n_1 * n_2 / m = 4064 * 1540 / 171 = 36{,}599$$
$$\text{number observed, } n, = a + b + c = 171 + 3893 + 1369 = 5433$$
$$\text{hidden, } x, = N - n, \text{ or, } c * b / a = 36{,}599 - 5433 \text{ or } 1369 * 3893 / 171 = 31{,}166$$
$$95\% \text{c.i.} = 1.96 * \sqrt{(n_1 * n_2 * b * c)/m^3} = 1.96 * \sqrt{(1540 * 4064 * 3893 * 1369)/171^3} = 4516$$
$$\text{Rounded Estimate of IU in Bangkok in 1991} = 36{,}600 \ (32{,}000 \text{ to } 40{,}800)$$

KEY
a or m = marks, number of people in both S1 and S2
b = number in S1 but not S2
c = number in S2 but not in S1
x = hidden population, number of people not in S1 or S2
n_1 = number of people in S1
n_2 = number of people in S2
N = total population

sources (i.e., the number of people that occur in more than one data source) is used to estimate the sampling intensity (i.e., the total proportion of injectors in the samples). These estimates of the number unobserved are then combined with the number in the data sources to generate the overall prevalence estimate. Studies with two samples can be easily calculated (see below). Those with three, four or more samples require statistical packages (such as STATA or GLIM or SPSS) as the data are analyzed using log-linear models with dependencies (technically, 'interactions') between data sources to generate an adjusted prevalence estimate. The following references give an essential background to the methods and their use in epidemiology (Hook and Regal, 1995; International Working Group for Disease Monitoring and Forecasting, 1995).

Case study 2a shows an example by Mastro and colleagues (1994) who carried out a two sample study in Bangkok in 1991. They collected two samples, 4064 heroin users in methadone treatment and 1540 people that had been arrested and tested positive for opiates. There were 171 people on both lists giving an estimate of 36,600 opiate users (0.5 percent of total population) in Bangkok in 1991.

Case Study 2b. Multi-data source Capture-recapture Study of Prevalence of IDU in Brighton, UK, 2001

Contingency Table—showing number of subjects matched between data sources

Brighton		*Treatment*							
		Yes				*No*			
		Arrest Referral							
		Yes		*No*		*Yes*		*No*	
		Survey & A&E							
		Yes	No	Yes	No	Yes	No	Yes	No
Syringe	Yes	1	8	7	65	3	19	36	521
Exchange	No	2	7	6	103	2	42	74	.

Data sources:

Specialist Drug Treatment	Arrest Referral	Survey & A&E	Syringe Exchange	Total records	Total Individuals	Matched	
199	84	131	660	1074	896	156	17%

Prevalence estimate:

population (15–44)	observed	estimate of unobserved	Total number IDU (95% CI)		Prevalence (95% CI)	
117,032	*896*	*1,408*	*2,304*	*1514–3737*	*2.0%*	*1.3–3.2%*

Model Selection:

Interactions: treatment*arrest referral, treatment *syringe exchange, arrest referral*survey_a&e syringe exchange*survey_a&e G^2 11.81, p-value 0.98, degrees of freedom 24

The problem with the two-sample study is that it is not known whether the two data sources (police and treatment) are independent (assumption #4). If not, and the proportion of the population captured or observed in the data sources is low (1 in 7 in the Bangkok study) then the potential for error is large (Wittes et al., 1974).

In a study in Brighton four data sources were analyzed (specialist drug treatment, criminal justice, syringe exchange, and community survey). The box (above) shows the contingency table, summary of the data sources, prevalence estimates and the best fitting model. The contingency table, instead of a 2 *2 as in the Bangkok study, shows the number of subjects across all four data sources. The number unobserved in the last cell with a "." represents those cases that do not appear on any of the data sources. In total 156 subjects (17 percent) were on more than one data source and one person was on all four data sources. The analysis suggested that the best model identified complex interactions between the data sources, making the basic analyses difficult and less reliable than if only a simple model was required for the data. The prevalence estimate itself could be considered high at 2 percent among adults aged 15–44. The authors note that compared to many capture-recapture studies for drug use the estimated number and proportion of unobserved subjects is comparatively low (i.e., ~900 : 1400, 1 : 1.5); that the capture-recapture estimate was lower than for a mortality multiplier estimate; and that local policy-makers were consulted and agreed that the estimate was consistent with other available information.

We should note here that complex dependency models can result from heterogeneity among the subjects (violation of assumption #2). Heterogeneity is often regarded as inevitable when using health data (Hook and Regal, 1995) as there are many examples of differences in health seeking behaviors and arrests by gender, age-group, social class, ethnic group, and degree of dependence. To avoid or limit the influence of these factors, analyses are made by first stratifying the data into more homogeneous subsets of people that are analyzed separately (for example, fitting separate models for males and females or by age group). Alternatively, co-variate capture-recapture techniques have been developed that allow fewer models to be fitted including both dependencies between data sources and those potentially between covariates (e.g., by gender and age-group) (Tilling and Sterne, 1999).

Two other assumptions that were potentially violated in this and many capture-recapture studies are *misclassification* bias (assumption #3) and closed population (assumption #1). Often there is insufficient information in the data sources to identify matching individuals; moreover subjects may give pseudonyms to different data sources to protect their identity. Studies would benefit by estimating the misclassification error thus allowing sensitivity tests of the robustness of the estimates (as animal ecology studies allow for loss of marks).

A *closed population* (i.e., no deaths, new cases, cessation or migration) is clearly an impossibility, but the bias of using an open capture-recapture method can be limited if the study time interval is short in comparison to the life cycle of the subject (e.g., a year for an injecting drug user may not be too serious a bias and allows sufficient data to be gathered to identify matches). Alternatively, open capture-recapture models seek to estimate population prevalence and change over time. However, there are very few examples of this approach in the epidemiological literature. One such study estimated the prevalence of street sex workers in Glasgow (McKeganey et al., 1992) through fieldwork over a succession of nights. They built "capture-histories" of women (e.g., on how many nights they were observed). The study suggested that the number of sex workers on the street remained approximately the same over a year but that the population of sex workers changed at approximately 8 percent per week. A new study by Kimber and colleagues used attendance histories at a safe injecting room to estimate prevalence over time (Jo Kimber, personal communication). This type of application is rare as there are hardly any single data sources that could meet assumption #2, requiring the data source to be representative of the target population. Pollack (1990) proposed mixed closed and open models as an answer to problems of heterogeneity, dependence, and dynamic populations, which may prove interesting to pilot in drug abuse.

2.3. Other Indirect Methods

Multiplier and capture-recapture estimates are the most common indirect prevalence methods used for problem drug use. Below, we mention other methods, some more recent in their development: truncated poisson, synthetic estimation, back calculation, and enhanced/event based multipliers.

2.3.1. Truncated Poisson

Truncated Poisson methods use information on repeat events to estimate the size of the population with 0 events. All the assumptions above apply, however, the strength of two of these assumptions and the availability of data limit its use. For instance, the assumption that repeat events are independent, i.e., that a person arrested or in treatment once is as likely to be re-arrested or re-enter treatment as someone who has not yet been "captured"; and the assumption that *all* subjects are as likely as each other to generate an event are easily violated. Also, as in the case of open capture-recapture models, the problem is to find a single data source that is representative of problem drug users. Certainly, criminal justice or specialist drug treatment data alone are not sufficient. Hay and Smit (2003) demonstrated the potential of truncated poisson applied to injecting drug users attending a syringe exchange in Scotland, estimating from attendance records of 647 subjects in a city in Scotland that there were a total of 1041 injectors.

2.3.2. Synthetic Estimation

Synthetic estimation or the multiple indicator method is a form of extrapolation (or technically 'regression on principal components'), which makes use of known prevalence figures in certain regions (that may have been estimated using multiplier or capture-recapture methods) to estimate prevalence in other regions. To do this correctly, these regions for which prevalence is being estimated must have data sources that are the same as (or very similar to) the regions for which prevalence estimates exist.

Extrapolation can be based on a single value, e.g., the proportion of opiate overdose deaths (Hall et al., 2000), or multiple indicators (Frischer 2001, Kraus 2003). It should be noted that there are some technical and statistical considerations that apply when more than one anchor point is used in a regression analysis, requiring discussion with an experienced statistician. For example, should a Poisson regression be used as opposed to using simple linear regression analysis and should rates or log-transformed data be used; should a weighting for the different anchor points be established to represent the reliability of the problem drug use prevalence estimate; and is the relationship between the drug indicator and the problem drug use prevalence rates similar across all the data points and is the relationship between prevalence and indicators valid.

2.3.3. Back-calculation

Law and colleagues (2001), and De Angelis and colleagues (in press) adapted back-calculation methods to estimate the incidence and prevalence of heroin use. The back-calculation method developed in AIDS epidemiology is based on the relationship between the time of infection (the presence of HIV), the incubation time, and the development of the disease (the diagnosis of AIDS). Knowledge of any two of these three components allows estimation of the third. Typically, the distribution of the incubation time and the incidence of the end point are assumed known and the infection process underlying the observed incidence is estimated. The estimated infection process is then used with the same information on the incubation time to predict the incidence and prevalence of the end-point of interest. When used for drug abuse epidemiology the observed incidence of the end-point has generally been opiate overdose death, with trends over time provided by routine mortality statistics. The "incubation" distribution is the distribution of the time between starting and stopping injecting, where the stopping process is the result of either a fatal overdose or the actual cessation of injecting. The data demands are considerable including reliable mortality statistics to identify the number of opiate overdose deaths, data on the opiate overdose and other drug related mortality rates of injecting drug users, and information on the cessation rates from injecting.

2.3.4. Enhanced/Event Based Multipliers

Simeone and colleagues (1997) have suggested modifications to the simple multiplier. Instead of a single proportion as a multiplier, a detailed multiple event history using multiple data sources are collected, in order theoretically to adjust for the inherent biases present in any single data source. However, these methods have only been piloted and are not in general use.

3. CONCLUSIONS

This chapter presented the indirect methods currently being used to estimate the prevalence of drug abuse in various populations. We have been critical of these methods pointing out their limitations and that the estimates derived from them need to be interpreted with caution. However, we believe that they are the answer to the problem of estimating the prevalence of rare problem drug using behaviors such as the use of heroin, drug injecting, or crack-cocaine use as population surveys are inefficient and not cost effective. Data sources for capture-recapture and multplier estimates should be carefully chosen to minimize both dependence and heterogeneity. Most communities have data that are available and these can be assessed for their utility for prevalence estimation. For example, do the data sources collect data on drug profile (injecting status, and problem drugs), collect identifiers to allow matching with other data sources /or/ if anonymised suffer little under-reporting; would problem drug users remember or recognise being captured by the data source, are only a sub-set of problem drug users captured by the data source; is it known how the data sources relate to other potential data sources. If the available data sources are poor—recommend steps to policy-makers (and data owners) to improve them for future estimation work. Collecting the data is the most time consuming part of prevalence estimation work. This work could be dramatically reduced if contributing to prevalence estimates was one of the objectives of routine data on problem drug use—such that a "public health surveillance" system of problem drug use was developed that specifically linked and integrated multiple data sources to allow prevalence estimation.

Finally, multiplier and capture-recapture estimation methods tend to be more reliable within discrete geographical locations in part to avoid heterogeneity (i.e., the relationship between the population of problem drug users and data sources is likely to vary from city to city), which has implications for public health surveillance and the design of studies.

REFERENCES

Andima, H., Krug, D., Bergner, L., Patrick, S., and Whitman, S. (1973). A prevalence estimation model of narcotics addiction in New York City. *American Journal of Epidemiology* 98, pp. 56–62.

Archibald, C.P., Jayaraman,G.C., Major, C., Patrick, D.M., Houston, S.M., and Sutherland, D. (2001). Estimating the size of hard-to-reach populations: a novel method using HIV testing data compared to other methods. *AIDS* 15 (suppl3), pp. S41–48.

Aust, R., Sharp, C. and Goulden C. (2002). *Prevalence of drug use: Key findings from the 2001/2002 British Crime Survey. Findings 182* Home Office Research, Development and Statistics Directorate, London, England.

Bargagli AM, Hickman M, Davoli M, Perucci CA, Schifano P, Buster M, Brugal T, Vicente J. (Forthcoming) Drug related mortality and its impact on adult mortality in eight European countries.

Begon, M. (1979). *Investigating Animal Abundance- Capture-Recapture for Biologists.* Edward Arnold, London, England.

Bello, P.Y. and Chene, G. (1997). A capture-recapture study to estimate the size of the addict population in Toulouse, France. In: European Monitoring Centre for Drugs and Drug Addiction (EMCDDA). *Scientific Monograph Series No. 1. Estimating the Prevalence of Problem Drug Use in Europe.* EMCDDA, Lisbon, Portugal, pp. 91–103.

Berkelman RL, Buehler JW. (1991) Surveillance. Chapter 11 pp. 161–176 In: Holland WW, Detels R, Knox G. (Eds.), Oxford Textbook of Public Health. 2nd Edition. Volume 2. Oxford: OUP.

Bishop, Y.M.M., Fienberg, S.E. and Holland, P.W. (1975). *Discrete Multivariate Analysis: Theory and Practice.* MIT Press, Cambridge, Massachusetts, US.

Brugha, R., Swan, A.V., Hayhurst, G.K., and Fallon, M.P. (1998). A drug misuser prevalence study in a rural English district. *European Journal of Public Health* 8, pp. 34–36.

Centers for Disease Control. (1988). *Guidelines for evaluating surveillance systems*. MMWR 37, p. S5.

Centers for Disease Control. (1992). *Proceedings of the 1992 International Symposium on Public Health Surveillance*. MMWR 41 Supplement, pp. 1–218.

Chandra Sekar C, Edwards Deming W. (1949). On a method of estimating birth and death rates and the extent of registration. *American Statistical Association Journal* pp. 101–115.

Comiskey, C.M. and Barry, J.M. (2001). A capture-recapture study of the prevalence and implications of opiate use in Dublin. *European Journal of Public Health* 11(2), pp.198–200.

Cormack, R.M. (1999). Problems with using capture-recapture in epidemiology: An example of a measles epidemic. *Journal of Clinical Epidemiology* 52, pp. 909–914.

De Angelis, D., Hickman, M., and Yang, S. (In press). Estimating long-term trends in the incidence and prevalence of opiate/injecting drug use and the number of ex-users: The use of back-calculation methods and opiate overdose deaths. *American Journal of Epidemiology*.

Domingo-Salvany, A., Hartnoll, R.L., Maguire, A., Brugal, M.T., Albertin, P., Cayla, J.A., Casabona, J. and Suelves, J.M. (1998). Analytical considerations in the use of capture-recapture to estimate prevalence: Case studies of the estimation of opiate use in the metropolitan area of Barcelona, Spain. *American Journal of Epidemiology* 148(8), pp. 732–740.

Domingo-Salvany, A., Hartnoll, R.L., Maguire, A., Suelves, J.M. and Anto, J.M. (1995). Use of capture-recapture to estimate the prevalence of opiate addiction in Barcelona, Spain, 1989. *American Journal of Epidemiology* 141, pp. 567–574.

Dupont, R.L. and Piemme, T.E. (1973). Estimation of the number of narcotic addicts in an urban area. *Medical Annals of the District of Columbia* 42, pp. 323–326.

Duque-Portugal, F., Martin, A. J., Taylor, R. and Ross, M.W. (1994). Mark-recapture estimates of injecting drug users in Sydney. *Australian Journal of Public Health* 18, pp. 201–204.

European Monitoring Centre for Drugs and Drug Addiction (EMCDDA). (1997). *Scientific Monograph Series No. 1. Estimating the Prevalence of Problem Drug Use in Europe*. EMCDDA, Lisbon, Portugal.

European Monitoring Centre for Drugs and Drug Addiction (EMCDDA). (2000). *EMCDDA Recommended Draft Technical Tools and Guidelines—Key Epidemiological Indicator: Prevalence Of Problem Drug Use*. EMCDDA, Lisbon, Portugal. Available at: http://www.emcdda.org/situation/themes/problem_drug_use.shtml.

Fienberg, S.E. (1992). Bibliography on capture-recapture modelling with application to census undercount adjustment. *Surveillance Methodology* 18, pp. 143–154.

Frank, B., Schmeidler, J., Johnson, B. and Lipton, D.S. (1978). Seeking truth in heroin indicators: the case of New York City. *Drug and Alcohol Dependence* 3, pp. 345–358.

Frischer, M., Hickman, M., Kraus, L., Mariani, F. and Wiessing, L. (2001). Comparison of different methods for estimating the prevalence of problematic drug misuse in Great Britain. *Addiction.* 96: 1465–1476.

GAP Toolkit Module 3. (2002). *Prevalence Estimation—Indirect Methods for Estimating the Size of the Drug Problem*. UNDCP, Vienna, Austria. (Editors: Taylor C. Hickman M.).

Gfroerer, J. and Brodsky, M. (1992). The incidence of illicit drug use in the United States, 1962–1989. *British Journal of Addiction* 87, pp. 1345–1351.

Godfrey, C., Eaton, G., McDougall, C. and Culyer, A. (2002). *The Economic and Social Costs of Class A Drug Use in England and Wales, 2000*. Home Office Research Study 249. Home Office Research, Development and Statistics Directorate, London, England.

Hall, W., Ross, J., Lynskey, M., Law, M. and Degenhardt, L. (2000). How many dependent heroin users are there in Australia? *Medical Journal of Australia* 173, pp. 528–531.

Hartnoll, R., Lewis, R., Mitcheson, M. and Bryer, S. (1985). Estimating the prevalence of opioid dependence. *The Lancet* 1(8422), pp. 203–205.

Hay, G. (2000). Capture-recapture estimates of drug misuse in urban and non-urban settings in the north east of Scotland. *Addiction* 95, pp. 1795–1803.

Hay, G. and Smit, F. (2003). Estimating the number of drug injectors from needle exchange data. *Addiction Research and Theory* 11, pp. 235–243.

Hay, G. and McKegany, N. (1996). Estimating the prevalence of drug misuse in Dundee, Scotland: an application of capture-recapture methods. *Journal of Epidemiology and Community Health* 50, pp. 469–472.

Hickman, M., Stimson, G., Howe, S., Farrell, M., Taylor, C., Cox, S., Harvey, J., Frischer, M. and Tilling, K. (1999). Estimating the prevalence of problem drug use in inner-London: A discussion of three capture-recapture studies. *Addiction* 94, pp. 1653–1662.

Hickman M, Taylor C, Chatterjee A, Degenhardt L, Frischer M, Hay G, Tilling K. (2003). Estimating drug prevalence: Review of methods with special reference to developing countries. *UN Bulletin on Narcotics*; LIV (1 and 2), pp. 15–32.

Hickman M., Higgins V., Hope V., Bellis M., Tilling K., Walker A., Henry J. (2004). Injecting drug use in Brighton, Liverpool, and London: best estimates of prevalence and coverage of public health indicators. *Journal of Epidemiology and Community Health* 58(9), pp. 766–771.

Hook, E.B. and Regal, R.R. (1995). Capture recapture methods in epidemiology: Methods and limitations. *Epidemiologic Reviews* 17, pp. 243–264.

Hser, Y-I., Anglin, M.D., Wickens, T.D., Brecht, M.L. and Homer, J. (1992). Techniques for the Estimation of Illicit Drug Use. *Prevalence: An Overview of Relevant Issues*. National Institute of Justice, Washington, D.C.

Hunt, L.G. (1977). Recent spread of heroin use in the United States. *American Journal of Public Health* 64, pp. 16–23.

International Working Group for Disease Monitoring and Forecasting. (1995). Capture-recapture and multiple record systems estimation I: History and theoretical development. *American Journal of Epidemiology* 142, pp. 1047–1057.

Kehoe, L., Hall, W. and Mant, A. (1992). Estimates of the number of injecting drug users in a defined area. *Australian Journal of Public Health* 16, pp. 232–237.

Kraus L., Augustin R., Frisher M., Kummler P., Uhl A., Wiessing L. (2003). Estimating prevalence of problem drug use at national level in countries of the European Union and Norway. *Addiction* 98, pp. 471–485.

Larson, A., Stevens, A., and Wardlaw, G. (1994). Indirect estimates of "hidden" populations: Capture-recapture methods to estimate the numbers of heroin users in the Australian Capital Territory. *Social Science and Medici*ne 39, pp. 823–831.

Law, M., Lynskey, M., Ross, J. and Hall, W. (2001). Back-projection estimates of the number of dependent heroin users in Australia. *Addiction* 96, pp. 433–443.

Lynskey, M., Degenhardt, L., Law, M.G., Ross, J. and Hall, W. (In press). Capture-recapture estimates of the number of individuals who are heroin dependent in New South Wales, Australia. *Substance Use and Misuse.*

Mastro, T.D., Kitayaporn, D., Weniger, B.G., Vanichseni, S., Laosunthron, V., Thongchai, U., Uneklabh, V., Vhoopanya, K. and Kimpakarnjanarat, K. (1994). Estimating the number of HIV-infected injection drug users in Bangkok: a capture-recapture method. *American Journal of Public Health* 84, pp. 1094–1099.

Maxwell, J.C. (2000). Methods for estimating the number of hard core drug users. *Substance Use and Misuse* 35, pp. 399–420.

McKeganey, N., Barnard, M., Leyland, A., Coote, I. and Follet, E. (1992). Female streetworking prostitution and HIV infection in Glasgow. *British Medical Journal* 305, pp. 801–804.

National Research Council. (2001). *Informing America's Policy on Illegal Drugs: What We Don't Know Keeps Hurting US*. Editors, Manski C., Pepper J., Petrie C. National Academy Press, Washington, D.C.

Parker, H., Bakx, K. and Newcombe R. (1988). *Living with Heroin.* Milton Keynes: Open University Press.

Pollack K.H., Nichols J.D., Brownie C., Hines J.E. (1990). Statistical inference for capture-recapture experiments, Wildlife Monographs, Wildlife Society, Department of Fisheries and Wildlife Sciencies, Virginia Polytechnic Institute and State University, Blacksburg, VA.

Rittenhouse, J.D. (Editor). (1977). *The Epidemiology of Heroin and Other Narcotics.* National Institute on Drug Abuse Research Monograph 16. National Institute on Drug Abuse, Rockville, Maryland.

Rhodes W. Synthetic estimation applied to the prevalence of drug use. (1993). *The Journal of Drug Issues* 23, pp. 297–321.

Seber, G.A.F. (1982). *The Estimation of Animal Abundance and Related Parameters.* 2nd Edition. Charles W Griffin, London, England.

Simeone, R., Rhodes, W., Hunt, D. and Truitt, L. (1997). *A Plan for Estimating the Number of "Hardcore" Drug Users in the United States.* Drug Policy Research Group, Office of National Drug Control Policy, Washington, D.C.

Squires, N.F., Beeching, N.J., Schlect, J.M. and Ruben, S.M. (1995). An estimate of the prevalence of drug misuse in Liverpool and a spatial analysis of known addiction. *Journal of Public Health and Medicine* 17(1), pp. 103–109.

Suzman, S., Sirken, M.G. and Cowan, C.D. (1988). Sampling rare and elusive populations. *Science* 240, pp. 991–996.

Tilling, K. and Sterne, J.A.C. (1999). Capture recapture models including covariate effects. *American Journal of Epidemiology* 149(4), pp. 392–400.

Wittes, J.T., Colton, T. and Sidel, V.W. (1974). Capture-recapture methods for assessing the completeness of case ascertainment when using multiple information sources. *Journal of Chronic Diseases* 27, pp. 25–36.

9

Qualitative Methods in the Drug Abuse Field

Claire E. Sterk and Kirk W. Elifson

1. INTRODUCTION

Drug use and abuse appear to be an integral part of our modern society and much emphasis is placed on identifying how many people use drugs, how often they use and what they use. Researchers, policymakers, service providers, the media and the public at large often highlight the social and health consequences of use, including the economic costs to individual users as well as society at

CLAIRE E. STERK • Emory University, Rollins School of Public Health
KIRK W. ELIFSON • Georgia State University, Department of Sociology

large. Trend data are used to show how the popularity of some drugs decreases, while that of others increases. Depending on the trends, policies are adjusted, monies are allocated for specific programs, research priorities are modified, and societal concerns shift. No consensus has been reached about which drugs to include in investigations. Some prefer the inclusion of any substance that can be abused. Others prefer to distinguish between legal drugs—e.g., prescription drugs, alcohol, and tobacco— and illegal drugs. Again others create a hierarchy among illegal drugs ranging from soft to hard drugs. No matter how long and detailed the list of drugs, the emergence of new drugs always needs to be considered.

Additional challenges emerge such as the definition and the operationalization of drug use and user. What constitutes a drug user? Is it a person who reports to have used drugs only once in his or her life or does the person need to have used more than once to be labeled a user? How about the person who did use drugs regularly but who has not used in the recent past which may be defined as the last five, three or one year? Among those identified as users, a wide variation in frequency and quantity of use may occur. For instance, what does it mean if a person indicates having used a substance four times during the past month as opposed to every day? Did the person use only one time during each intake or did each use session include multiple use events? Was the amount taken each time the same? Was the quality of the drug similar during all occasions? Did the user simultaneously use other drugs or use other drugs immediately before of after using this drug?

The quest for knowledge among social scientists emphasizes a sound measure of drug use from a socio-cultural perspective. Methodological pluralism often characterizes such research and the two main paradigms are quantitative and qualitative research. Quantitative researchers, for instance, value a reliable assessment of the prevalence and incidence of use by population group and pattern. Their qualitative peers, on the other hand, primarily focus on the impact of the context on use patterns and the meaning of drug intake to the users themselves (Sterk, 2004). The epidemiological paradigm is grounded in a positivist scientific approach that emphasizes scientific objectivity and the ultimate outcome of measuring "reality." In other words, the findings from such studies are neither empirically nor conceptually related to the social context. The qualitative paradigm, on the other hand, emphasizes the importance of a holistic understanding of all phenomena involved, thereby requiring an emphasis on behaviors in their natural setting and exploratory narratives provided by members of the group under study. "Objectivity" is not only determined by the researchers but also by the study participants and commonly the scientific rigor is expected to lead to findings in which all parties are aware of their assumptions. This contradicts the underlying assumption in epidemiological inquiries that the investigators *a priori* determine what questions are relevant (for more detail see Sterk and Elifson, 2004). The differences between the epidemiological and qualitative research paradigm also are revealed in the data analysis process (Creswell, 1994; Guba and Lincoln,

1988). Epidemiological studies produce numerical data and the analysis process focuses on statistical correlations, predictions, and significance. Qualitative studies produce textual data and the analysis process focuses on identifying salient themes that provide an interpretative understanding, thereby allowing for bridging population-based data to individual variance and meaning. In general, quantitative epidemiological methods build on the deductive logic in which the research design lacks flexibility. Whereas qualitative methods build on the inductive logic in which the research design is dynamic and emerges as the study evolves. Epidemiological findings assume reliability and validity as opposed to the validity and triangulation as highlighted in qualitative inquiries. The most comprehensive insights of drug use clearly can be acquired when combining the quantitative and qualitative research paradigms

1.1. Qualitative Inquiries of Drug Use

Among drug researchers, ethnography has a longstanding tradition. Among the earliest examples from the United States are *The Road to H.* (Chein et al., 1964), *Portraits from a Shooting Gallery* (Fiddle, 1967), and *Taking Care of Business: The Heroin User's Life on the Street* (Prebble and Casey, 1969). In the 1970s, Agar (1973) focused on the language used among heroin users as reported in *Ripping and Running: A Formal Ethnography of Urban Heroin Addicts.* Other studies emphasize the unique features of drug using life styles such as in *Careers in Dope* (Waldorf, 1973), *Shooting Dope: Career Patterns of Hard-Core Heroin Users* (Faupel, 1991), *Cocaine Changes: The Experience of Using and Quitting* (Waldorf, Reinarman, and Murphy, 1991) and *Tricking and Tripping: Prostitution in the AIDS Era* (Sterk, 2000).

These and other studies have made significant contributions to our understanding of the lives of users, including the various social roles and associated behaviors (Bourgeois, 1989; Stephens, 1991), the unique experiences of female drug users (Rosenbaum, 1981; Sterk, 1999; Taylor, 1993), and the link with the underground economy (Maher, 1997). Like all ethnographies, those in the drug field are a product of their time. For example, it is no coincidence that up until the 1980s, most research focused on heroin, the "drug of choice" during that era. During the 1980s and 1990s, heroin was replaced by crack cocaine and more recently by methamphetamine, ecstasy and other club drugs.

Qualitative studies of drug use often are disregarded and dominance of textual versus numerical data is viewed as a weakness. This is reflected in comments that label qualitative data as anecdotal information. Qualitative studies are faulted for the typically small sample size, the active involvement of the researcher in the data collection process, the flexibility in selecting topics to be discussed in interviews, and the labor-intensive processes involving data analysis. Critics often ignore the foundations of qualitative research including the fact that generalizibility is not a goal and that the involvement of the researcher always occurs when collecting information and that the more collaborative role of qualitative researchers is assumed in order to allow for discoveries that are difficult to make during more quantitative "interrogations." Furthermore, questionnaires may miss salient dimensions even though the data suggest statistically significant findings, and that quantitative research is time consuming during the earlier stages of the process when hypotheses are formulated, sampling frames are determined, and questionnaires are constructed and tested. What follows is an introduction to the qualitative research paradigm, including a presentation of the main data collection methods.

2.   QUALITATIVE RESEARCH: BACKGROUND OVERVIEW

Prior to discussing qualitative research that focuses on drug use, a brief history on the method will be presented. When reviewing the epistemology, style and ethics of qualitative inquiries, one can distinguish seven historical periods (Denzin and Lincoln, 2000). These periods include the traditional period (1900–1950) during which qualitative researchers tended to use positivist approaches to produce "objective" accounts of exotic cultures (Geertz, 1988; Rosaldo, 1989); the modernist period (1950–1970) during which emphasis was placed on formalizing qualitative research as well as its use in gaining an understanding of social processes (Taylor and Bogdan, 1998; Glaser and Strauss, 1967; Lofland and Lofland, 1995); the blurred genres period (1970–1986) focused on representation and the search among qualitative researchers to locate themselves and their subjects in reflexive text (Geertz, 1973; 1983). The distinction between the social sciences and humanities became blurred during this later period. The crisis of the representation period (1986–1990) was characterized by the search for new models of truth, method and representation and the writing become increasingly reflective (Clough, 1992; Rosaldo, 1989). This perspective extended into the post-modern period (1990–1995) of experimental ethnographic writing and the post-experimental inquiry (1995–present).

In this chapter, we will use the following definition of qualitative research: "qualitative research is a situated activity that locates the observer in the world. It consists of a set of interpretive, material practices that make the world visible. These practices . . . turn the world into a series of representations, including field notes, interviews, conversations, photographs, recordings, and memos to the self. At this level, qualitative research involves an interpretive, naturalistic approach to the world" (Denzin and Lincoln, 2000). Qualitative researchers have been compared with "quilt makers," researchers who assemble information into salient themes that result in a holistic picture from an insider's perspective (Becker, 1998). The most common data collection strategies in drug research (interviewing, focus groups, and observation) will be presented below.

2.1. Interviewing

Interviewing can include face-to-face individual, dyadic or group interviewing, and telephone or web-based surveys. Interviews can be informal and unstructured or more formal and semi-structured or structured. Finally, interviews can involve a one-time event or a series of data collection moments (see, for example, Lincoln and Guba, 1985; Spradley, 1979). The main goal of conducting an interview is for the interviewer to gain knowledge and insight from the respondent. Independent of the use of a quantitative or qualitative inquiry strategy, the interviewer has to be an "interested listener" who does not bias or judge the interviewees' responses (Converse and Schuman, 1974). This is especially important when interviewing drug users. They are enrolled in a study because they engage in an illegal behavior and they are being asked questions about this behavior, including associated actions such as involvement in criminal activities. If the respondent feels judged by the interviewer, the chances of collecting accurate information are reduced.

2.1.1.   Quantitative Versus Qualitative Interviews

The most common form of interviewing varies by research paradigm. In quantitative, including epidemiological, research structured interviews are most common. The researchers determine in advance which questions will be posed and which response categories are provided. The inclusion of the choice "other," acknowledges that the study participant may wish to provide an answer other than the options provided by the researchers. For example, in a face-to-face interview in which the interviewer records the answer, the interviewer reads the question, the respondent replies, and the interviewer records the response. There is no room for explanation, elaborations or conversation beyond the question and its response choices. The most common forms of interviewing in qualitative research are semi-structured and unstructured interviews. The assumption underlying semi-structured and unstructured interviewing is that the study participants are knowledgeable and offer a meaningful perspective. Consequently, the nature of the interaction between the interviewer and study participant is such that the interviewer seeks to establish rapport with the respondent and becomes an active participant. When conducting interviews with drug users, the user serves as the expert. Nevertheless, it is important that the interviewer be knowledgeable to ensure the respondent elaborates and provides adequate detail if an uncommon behavior is mentioned.

The semi-structured interview follows a series of open-ended questions that often are asked in a predetermined order. Unstructured interviews are centered around a series of open-ended questions or a list of topics to be discussed. The order in which topics are addressed is irrelevant and not all topics may be addressed

with each respondent. Unstructured interviewing also is guided by a set of pre-
determined topics, but the conversation—the data gathering process—determines
how and when in the dialogue the information is obtained. The results of unstructured and semi-structured interviews provide information on the topics and themes
that are salient to the study participant, the appropriate language to be used and the
meaning of this language, and the various sub-groups within the study population,
which in turn guide the recruitment strategies as well as the sampling frame. In
addition, this type of interviewing allows the interviewer to generate theory.

A unique form of qualitative interviews is the life history (Schwandt, 1997).
Life histories can include oral histories, autobiography, or life stories (Tierney,
1998). Life histories have the potential to provide a longitudinal perspective. For
example, in our study on intergenerational drug use, the life course perspective
allowed us to explore the impact of early household conditions, the influence of
parents and siblings, and the role of main life events of drug use (Sterk et al., 2003).

Qualitative interviews are more difficult to conduct than structured interviews
because the interviewer must constantly consider the participant's response and
probe for additional information. Probing is done by asking "directive questions"
about a specific topic or comment, repeating the last sentence of the answer,
summarizing the answer, or non-verbal expressions such as when the interviewer
nods his or her head, verbally through affirmative noises such as "uh-huh," "yeah,"
or "right," or being silent. A few moments of silence signal the expectation of
further elaboration and allow the respondent time for reflection, especially when
contemplating complex questions. It is through probing that the power differential
between the interviewer and the study participant is symbolized, even though the
conversation may appear to be one of equals.

2.2. Focus Groups

The most common form of a group interview is the focus group, an interview
in which a small group of people discusses a limited number of specific topics
during a one to two hour session. This type of qualitative data gathering involves
the simultaneous interviewing of individuals, whereby the emphasis is not on the
individual responses but on the interaction between the participants. The ideal size
of a focus group ranges between six and twelve individuals and the interviewer
is referred to as the moderator. Commonly, the participants are a homogeneous
group of individuals who do not know each other (Krueger, 1994). Focus groups as
an inquiry strategy emphasize the interaction between the group members rather
than the individual perspective (Merton, Riske and Kendall, 1956). The goal of
focus groups is not to reach a consensus. Instead, the aim is for the participants
to reflect on the discussion topics, to present their opinions, and to respond to the
comments of other group members. In other words, the focus is on the synergistic
group effect (Stewart and Shamdasani, 1990). When conducting focus groups on
drug use, it may be important to have separate groups depending on the drugs

people use or the ways in which they support their habit. For instance, it might be useful to have a focus group consisting only of women who trade sex for drugs. Too much heterogeneity among focus group participants may stand in the way of data collection in that a meaningful dialogue may be impeded.

The collective brainstorming process among focus group participants is disrupted if a group member dominates the discussion and a major challenge to the moderator is to ensure all voices are heard and to prevent distortion of individual opinions due to perceived group pressures. Another challenge encountered by researchers using focus groups is confidentiality. While the moderator can ensure confidentiality between him or herself and the participants, confidentiality among the participants is more difficult to guarantee. Increasingly, the latter is being emphasized in consent forms and a presentation of pre-focus group guidelines. The assumption sometimes is made that focus groups are very cost effective and require less time than individual qualitative interviews. However, one should keep in mind that these data collection strategies serve a unique purpose and provide different data. For example, focus group data reveal group dynamics and collective thinking, whereas individual interviews provide in-depth information from a single perspective. In a controlled experiment, Fern (1982) found that focus groups did not produce significantly more information that in-depth interviews. On the other hand, some research has shown that the participation in a group might be perceived as more satisfying and stimulating and less threatening than individual face-to-face interviews by the participants (Morgan, 1998; Wilkinson, 1998).

2.3. Observations

While much of the emphasis in interviewing is on what people say, observations focus on what people do. Observational techniques largely are part of the qualitative paradigm, but even quantitative investigators may rely to a limited extent on observations. For example, during a street interview non-verbal responses and comments on the interviewee's actions and gestures may be recorded. In order to observe, the researcher has to be part of the setting and much of the ongoing debate has focused on the question to what extent this presence may change the situation under study (see, for example, Adler and Adler, 1986). The least involved method of observations involves "windshield observations" in which the researcher is only marginally involved.

When conducting observations, researchers must attend to their role and the extent to which they will immerse themselves in the group under study. The level of involvement can range from being a "distant" observer to a "complete" participant. Others have referred to this as a spectrum of membership roles, including "peripheral" or "active" and "complete" members. Clearly these distinctions are related to discussions about the reliability and validity of observation data. When studying drug users, the observer should take caution in terms his or her own safety but also the safety of others. Again others are less concerned with the observer's role but more with developing a typology of systematic observations, consisting of descriptive, focused and selective observations (Werner and Schoepfle, 1987). Observation as an inquiry strategy also has been referred to as ethnography or fieldwork. The process of conducting observations has been labeled as "subjective soaking" (Ellen, 1984) and the written analysis has been referred to as "thick description" (Geertz, 1973).

In order to be able to observe, the researcher has to identify appropriate settings as well as strategies to gain entrance to these settings (Lincoln and Guba, 1985). Ethnographic mapping is ideally suited to make initial decisions about potential study settings, especially since such mapping involves the recording of the physical as well as the social infrastructure of these settings (Sterk, 1999). Public settings are clearly less difficult to enter than private settings. In addition, researchers can more easily conduct observations in public than in private settings. As a result, much of the debate on observation research in public settings and among vulnerable populations has centered on the ethics surrounding "covert" observations.

Once settings have been identified and access has been mediated, the researcher will have developed some contacts with the "gatekeepers." In public settings these are more difficult to identify than in private settings. Gatekeepers may assist the researcher in gaining entry, may prevent entry, or may bias the process to guide the researcher to only certain segments of the setting or population under study. Situations with multiple gatekeepers may require diplomacy to avoid aligning too closely with certain persons or segments. Ideally, the observer should connect with gatekeepers who are guides as well as informants (Sterk, 2000). The mapping and negotiations with gatekeepers allow for the development of the observer's network and as the network expands the researcher is likely to become less dependent on her or his initial contacts. The emphasis shifts to building relationships and rapport, while observing and listening, becoming more focused, and writing extensive observation notes. Clearly, an effective observer is not a silent partner, but rather engages in many informal conversations with members of the group under study. Records of these conversations also become part of the records, often referred to as field notes. The writing of such notes requires specific skills and timing (for more information see Bernard, 1994; Sanjek, 1990). Overall, observation allows the researcher to collect data that are less based on reactivity than, for example interview data, it assists in identifying salient research questions, and helps provide insight into the social context in which people operate.

2.4.   Combining Multiple Data Collection Techniques and Triangulation

It is common for researchers to apply more than one data collection strategy. Examples of combinations involving interviews and focus groups are initial exploratory focus groups that allow for the identification of salient themes, followed by in-depth interviews or in-depth interviews followed by confirmatory focus groups. Combining observations and interviews is commonly done as well, with some initiating the observations prior to the interviews as a means to learn about settings, sub-populations, and other characteristics of the study population and others conducting the observations and interviews simultaneously. Finally, there are scenarios that involve all three data collection methods. Moreover, the combined use of methods also may include archival and historical inquiries and quantitative data collection. The latter may involve surveys that are preceded or followed by focus groups, interviews that are a combination of questionnaire-based and open-ended questions, and surveys that include extensive mapping and observations.

The value of combining various data collection methods is that it allows for comprehensive data. In methodological terms, the use of multiple methods is referred to as triangulation (Denzin, 1989). Triangulation allows the researcher to capture the multiple realities, including the researcher's experiences in qualitative investigations. Drug use is such a complex phenomenon that the use of multiple methods increases the likelihood of adequately capturing all dimensions. More recently, the concept of "crystallization" has been introduced (Richardson, 2003). Whereas triangulation assumes that there is a fixed domain for which comparisons can be made, crystallization assumes more complexity and emphasizes that any researcher's findings are determined by the angle (of the crystal) or perspective of the individual, including the study participants.

A core concept among drug abuse researchers is that of a "primary drug of choice." The use of multiple methods and subsequent triangulation can assist in an understanding of how drug users specify this drug, a dimension that often is missing especially in quantitative investigations. Measures of consumption in the form of counts of number of drugs used or type of drug used by frequency do not capture the fact that users of multiple substances frequently prefer some drug(s) more than others and that these preferences may shift over time. In our own work we learned that drug users determined their primary drug of choices based on a number of criteria. These included the drug they were using most frequently at the time of the interview, their perception of which drug was most prevalent on the local drug market, their ideas of the eligibility criteria for the study, the reputation of the drug in society at large, and the legal repercussions for its use. For example, users mentioned cocaine as their drug of choice but in the in-depth interviews they expressed that they preferred methamphetamine over cocaine; users listed crack as their drug of choice because of its availability and the lack of availability of high quality heroin which was their drug of choice; users did not mention crack as their drug of choice because of its negative reputation; while others mentioned marijuana as their primary drug of choice because the legal repercussions were modest compared to those faced by crack users. Through observations we learned that people who listed a drug of choice never used that drug because of its lack of availability. In focus groups we learned that users do not mention certain drugs as their primary choice because of the negative associations.

3. CONCLUDING REMARKS

Qualitative researchers have made major contributions to the drug abuse field. It is an ideal research paradigm for inquiries on complex phenomena. Unfortunately, quantitative and qualitative research approaches are perceived as irreconcilable. In reality, however, both types of researchers aim to gain an understanding of the people under study and they do so by interpreting the data. The difference may be that quantitative researchers interpret the numbers, whereas qualitative researchers interpret narratives. Nevertheless, interpretation is essential in both approaches. Distinctions in methodological issues certainly exist but instead of focusing on the weaknesses of each, the substance abuse field can gain from building on the strengths of each paradigm.

Rapid qualitative assessments also have been recognized as valuable when epidemiological indicators are unavailable. In addition to serving as a substitute for quantitative data in countries that lack an epidemiological tradition, rapid assessments also are used in settings where such data are available. In the latter case, the rapid assessment serves the purpose of providing information on specific subgroups and settings (Scrimshaw, Carbello, and Ramos, 1991; Stimson, Fitch and Rhodes, 1999; Trotter et al., 2001).

REFERENCES

Adler, P.A. and Adler, P. (1986). *Membership Roles In Field Research*. Sage Publications, Beverly Hills, CA.

Agar, M. (1973). *Ripping and Running: A Formal Ethnography of Urban Heroin Users*. Academic Press, New York.

Becker, H.S. (1998). *Tricks of the Trade: How to Think about Your Research While You're Doing It*. University of Chicago Press, Chicago.

Bernard, H.R. (1994). *Research Methods in Anthropology: Qualitative And Quantitative Approaches*. (2nd edition). Alta Mira, Walnut Creek, CA.

Bourgois, P. (1995). *In Search of Respect: Selling Crack in El Barrio*. Cambridge University Press, New York.

Chein, I., Gerard, D., Lee, R. and Rosenfeld. E. (1964). *The Road to H.: Narcotics, Juvenile Delinquency, and Social Policy*. Basic Books, New York.

Clough, P.T. (1992). *The End(S) of Ethnography: From Realism To Social Criticism*. (2nd edition). Peter Lang, New York.

Converse, J.M. & Schuman, H. (1974). *Conversations at Random: Survey Research as Interviewers See It*. John Wiley, New York.

Creswell, J.W. (1994). *Research Design: Qualitative and Quantitative Approaches*. Sage Publications, Thousand Oaks, CA.

Denzin, N.K. (1989). *Interpretive Biography*. Sage Publications, Newbury Park, CA.

Denzin, N., and Lincoln, Y. (2000). *Handbook of Qualitative Research*. Sage Publications, Newbury Park, CA.

Ellen, R.F. (1984). *Ethnographic Research*. Academic Press, New York.

Faupel, C. (1991). *Shooting Dope: Career Patterns of Hard-Core Heroin Users* University of Florida Press, Gainesville, FL.

Fern, R.N. (1982). The use of focus groups for idea generation: The effects of group size, acquaintanceship, and moderator on a response quality and quantity. *Journal of Marketing Research* 19, pp. 1–13.

Fiddle, S. (1967). *Portraits from a Shooting Gallery*. Harper and Row, New York.

Geertz, C. (1973). *The Interpretation of Cultures: Selected Essays*. Basic Books, New York.

Geertz, C. (1983). *Local Knowledge: Further Essays in Interpretive Anthropology*. Basic Books, New York.

Geertz, C. (1988). *Works and Lives: The Anthropologist as Author*. Stanford University Press, Stanford, CA.

Glaser, B., and Strauss, A. (1967). *The Discovery Of Grounded Theory: Strategies For Qualitative Research*. Aldine de Gruyter, New York.

Guba, E.G. & Lincoln, Y. (1988). Do inquiry paradigms imply inquiry methodologies? In: Fetterman, D.M. (Ed.), *Qualitative Approaches to Evaluation in Education*, Praeger, New York. pp. 88–115.

Krueger, R.A. (1994). *Focus Groups: A Practical Guide For Applied Research*. (2nd edition). Sage Publications, Thousand Oaks, CA.

Lincoln, Y.S. & Guba, E.G. (1985). *Naturalistic Inquiry*. Sage Publications, Beverly Hills, CA.

Lofland, J. and Lofland, L.H. (1995). *Analyzing Social Settings: A Guide to Qualitative Observation and Analysis*. (3rd Edition). Wadworth, Belmont, CA.

Maher, L. (1997). *Sexed Work: Gender, Race And Resistance In A Brooklyn Drug Market*. Oxford University Press, Oxford.

Merton, R., Riske, M. & Kendall, P.L. (1956). *The Focused Interview*. Free Press, New York.

Morgan, D.L. (1998). *The Focus Group Guide Book*. Sage Publications, New York.

Prebble, E., and Casey, J. (1969). Taking Care of Business: the heroin user's life on the street. *The International Journal of the Addictions* 4, pp. 1–24.

Richardson, L. (2003). *Writing: A method of inquiry*. In: Denzin, N, and Lincoln, Y. (Eds.), *Collecting and Interpreting Qualitative Materials*. (2nd edition). Sage Publications, Thousand Oaks, CA.

Rosaldo, R. (1989). *Culture And Truth: The Remaking Of Social Analysis*. Beacon Press, Boston.

Rosenbaum, M. (1981). *Women on Heroin*. Rutgers University Press, New Brunswick, NJ.

Sanjek, R. (1990). *Fieldnotes*. Cornell University Press, Ithaca.

Schwandt, T.A. (1997). *Qualitative Inquiry: A Dictionary of Terms*. Sage Publications, Thousand Oaks, CA.

Scrimshaw, S.C.M., Carballo, M. and Ramos, L., (1991). The AIDS rapid anthropological assessment procedures: A tool for health education planning and evaluation. *Health Education Quarterly* 18(1), pp. 111–123.

Spradley, J.P. (1979). *The Ethnographic Interview*. Holt, Rinehart and Winston, New York.

Stephens, R. (1991). *The Street Addict Role*. State University of New York Press, Albany.

Sterk, C. (1999). *Fast Lives: Women Who Use Crack Cocaine*. Temple University Press, Philadelphia.

Sterk, C. (2000). *Tricking and Tripping: Prostitution During the AIDS Era*. Social Change Press, Putnam Valley, NY.

Sterk, C. (2004). *The "Substances" In Addiction: Socially Constructed or Scientifically Determined?* Emory University Press, Atlanta, GA.

Sterk, C. and Elifson, K. (2004). Qualitative methods in community-based research. In: Blumenthal, D., and DiClemente, R. (Eds.), *Community Based Health Research*, Springer, New York. pp. 189–219.

Sterk, C., Elifson, K., Wilson, K., and Mills, M. (2003). *Cocaine use, trajectories and mental health: parental and sibling influences*. Paper presented at the Annual Meeting of the Society for Social Problems, Atlanta, GA.

Sterk, C., Dolan, K. Hatch, S. (1999). Epidemiological indicators and ethnographic realities of female cocaine use. *Journal of Substance Abuse and Use* 34(14):2057–2072.

Stimson, G., Fitch, C. and Rhodes, T. (Eds.), (1999). *The Rapid Assessment and Response Guide on Psychoactive Substance Use and Prevention* (PSUP-RAR). World Health Organization Programme on Substance Abuse and UNAIDS, UNDCP, UNICEF, Geneva.

Taylor, A. (1993). *Women Drug Users: An Ethnography of a Female Injecting Community*. Claridon Press, Oxford.

Taylor, S.J. & Bogdan, R. (1998). *Introduction to qualitative research methods: A guidebook and resource*. New York: John Wiley.

Tierney, W.G. (1998). Life history's history: Subjects foretold. *Qualitative Inquiry* 4, pp. 49–70.

Trotter, R., Needle, R., Goosby, E., Bates, C., and Singer M. (2001). A methodological model for rapid assessment, response, and evaluation: The RARE program in public health. Field Methods 13(2), pp. 137–159.

Waldorf, D. (1973). *Careers in Dope*. Englewood Cliffs (NJ): Prentice Hall.

Waldorf, D., Reinarman, C., and Murphy, S. (1991). *Cocaine Changes: The Experience of Using and Quitting*. Temple University Press, Philadelphia.

Werner, O. & Schoepfle, G.M. (1987). *Systematic Fieldwork: Vol. 1. Foundations Of Ethnography And Interviewing*. Sage Publications, Newbury Park, CA.

Wilkinson, S. (1998). Focus groups in feminist research: Power, interaction, and the co-construction of meaning. *Women's Studies International Forum* 21, pp. 111–125.

10

Ethical Considerations for Drug Abuse Epidemiologic Research

Craig L. Fry and Wayne Hall

CRAIG L. FRY • Turning Point Alcohol and Drug Centre, Melbourne, Australia and Fellow, Department of Public Health, University of Melbourne
WAYNE HALL • Director, Office of Public Policy and Ethics, Institute for Molecular Bioscience, University of Queensland

1. EPIDEMIOLOGY, DRUGS AND ETHICS

The mortality and morbidity caused by alcohol, tobacco and illicit drug misuse represents a significant public health burden (Ezzati et al., 2002). A key part of the public health response is the collection of epidemiological and social science data to define at-risk populations to identify opportunities for intervention and to evaluate the effectiveness of policies in preventing or treating drug misuse and drug-related harm. The systematic use of epidemiological and social science research methods to study illicit drug use is barely 40 years old in the United States and United Kingdom, which have pioneered this approach. Because of the sensitive nature of epidemiological research on illicit drug use a unique set of ethical challenges need to be explicitly addressed by the field. Although ethics guidelines have been proposed (Council for International Organizations of Medical Sciences, 1991), scholarship on the ethics of epidemiology is scant, and consensus on core values not yet achieved (Coughlin, 2000).

1.1. The Nature of Epidemiological Research on Drug Use

Epidemiological research on drug use includes: community surveys of licit and illicit drug use patterns that define populations at risk (Bachman et al., 1997); longitudinal studies of personal and social factors that predict the course of drug use (Bachman et al., 1997; Kandel and Chen, 2000; Wills et al., herein); studies of the prevalence and correlates of drug dependence in the general population using standardized diagnostic interviews (Anthony and Helzer, 1991); and observational studies of treated populations using administrative and health record systems to examine mortality, morbidity and abstinence rates among drug dependent persons (Hser et al., 2001). In the past decade drug epidemiology has increasingly applied a mix of quantitative and qualitative social research methods (see Rhodes et al., 2000). Methods developed by ethnographers have also been employed successfully in epidemiological studies of drug use (e.g. Agar, 1996; Maher et al., 1998).

Epidemiological drug research occurs in a variety of settings (e.g. schools, work place, public settings, prisons, drug treatment facilities etc), and includes diverse target groups (e.g. youth, sex workers, homeless people, homosexual men, indigenous peoples etc). The development of epidemiological research methods to study drug use has largely occurred in industrialized societies that have had substantial problems with illicit drug use in large cities and the societal resources to devote to studying this phenomenon. As the morbidity and mortality associated with illicit drug use has become internationally recognized, so too the application of epidemiological research methods has become increasingly global, extending frequently to developing countries.

The spread of such research beyond the settings in which it originated has in turn raised questions about the possible role of ethical frameworks that differ from those that have grown from the Western biomedical tradition. Resolving such questions will be important for successful international collaborations in drug epidemiology. For epidemiologists, an awareness of "alternative ethical arguments has become as important as knowing the advantages and disadvantages of different epidemiological techniques" (Roberts and Reich, 2002 p. 1059).

1.2. Why is Ethics Important in Drug Use Epidemiology?

Since the end of the Second World War, the world has witnessed the adverse effects of unethical experimentation on vulnerable groups using invasive medical interventions (Nazi medical experimentation, the Tuskegee syphilis study, clinical trial deaths etc) (Brody, 1998). These events prompted the development of international ethics guidelines for medical research with humans. Institutional ethics committee frameworks for the oversight and regulation of such research have also emerged in most developed countries to protect the rights of participants in medical research. These are enforced through obligatory compliance with the World Medical Association Declaration of Helsinki (see http://www.wma.net), or local frameworks that are consistent with the Helsinki principles.

The conduct of drug use epidemiology differs from traditional biomedical research in that it rarely involves invasive medical interventions that may directly harm or benefit study participants. Rather, it typically involves collection of sensitive personal information on drug use and illegal activities from study participants, where the principal potential harms arise if this information becomes known to third parties and used to the detriment of research participants (e.g. workplace discrimination, criminal prosecution). Participants in epidemiological research need to be protected from these outcomes. Discussions about the ethics of drug epidemiology connect closely with civil liberties, human rights and justice.

There are also compelling non-ethical reasons for protecting the confidentiality of drug research participants. Those who do participate in studies where confidentiality and other risks exist may be less forthcoming or even deliberately misleading about their drug use and related issues. Reliable and valid data on drug use requires well-designed epidemiological research that is conducted in accordance with accepted ethical standards.

2.   ETHICAL PRINCIPLES

There is little consensus among ethicists on the most appropriate approach to use in deciding how we should act in difficult cases (Beauchamp and Childress, 2001; Rachels, 1993). Among the competing ethical theories is "utilitarianism" which judges individual actions or moral rules according to their consequences (e.g. Singer, 1993), and "deontological" or duty-based ethical theories that propose that our actions should be guided by broad ethical principles or duties (e.g. Rawls, 1971). For a review of ethical theories refer to LaFollette (2001).

A number of ethical principles have been suggested as a form of common moral ground that can be accepted by most people. These include autonomy, beneficence and others that are discussed below. These principles alert us to the existence of important ethical issues but they alone do not solve our ethical problems or necessarily tell us how to behave. Making decisions about what is ethical behavior or processes requires more than simply following accepted prescriptions and principles (Jonsen, 1998). If we are to take a rule-based approach to ethics, these principles must be applied and tested in specific cases by a process of debate and discussion. This approach to applied ethical analysis is a useful starting point to develop ethical standards in drug epidemiology.

2.1.   Autonomy, Non-Maleficence, Beneficence, Justice

An influential set of moral principles has emerged from ethical analyses of biomedical research in the US (grounded in a Judaeo-Christian tradition of rule-based morality). These are the principles of autonomy, non-maleficence, beneficence, and justice (Beauchamp and Childress, 2001) that were originally derived from internationally recognized guidelines for the ethical conduct of medical research with humans (Brody, 1998; Beauchamp and Childress, 2001) but have been increasingly applied to all types of research with humans, including social and behavioral and epidemiological research.

Respect for autonomy means that we respect and not interfere with the actions of rational persons, persons who are assumed to be able to freely decide upon a course of action without being coerced or forced. In biomedical research, respect for autonomy requires that research participants give informed and voluntary consent to participate in research; that assurances are provided that the confidentiality and privacy of any personal information that they provide will be respected, and that researchers will be truthful about risks that may arise from their study participation (Beauchamp and Childress, 2001).

Non-maleficence simply means, "do no harm", and requires us to refrain from causing harm or injury, or from placing others at risk of harm or injury. In biomedical research, the principle requires researchers to minimize the risks of research participation (Brody, 1998; Beauchamp and Childress, 2001). Truth telling is also relevant to the principle of non-maleficence. Beneficence requires that research studies have a reasonable chance of producing benefits, and that the benefits of research outweigh any burdens or risks of participation. In biomedical research, this means not only that the benefits of the research to society outweigh the risks but also that the risks for individual participants are outweighed by the benefits of their participation.

The principle of distributive justice requires a fair and equitable distribution of the burdens and the benefits of research participation (Brody, 1998). This requires: that the risks of research participation were not unfairly distributed (e.g. confined to the poor and indigent); and that any benefits of research participation (e.g. access to promising new treatments) were fairly shared between all who potentially may benefit from it.

2.2. Ethical Requirements of Human Biomedical Research

Debate over the past half century about the applied ethics of medical research has produced a consensus on basic requirements for ethical biomedical research with human subjects (Brody, 1998; Jonsen, 1998). While conditions for ethical approval may differ in detail from country to country, the following basic set of ethical requirements or rules is found in most national guidelines (Brody, 1998).

2.2.1. Independent Ethical Review of Risks and Benefits

Before any human research proceeds, investigators must obtain ethical approval from an independent committee of ethical review. This is usually an Institutional Ethics Committee, although terminology differs between countries (e.g. Institutional Review Boards in the US, Human Research Ethics Committees in Australia etc), as do the ways in which these committees are constituted and how they operate. Their major aim is to provide an external and independent assessment of whether the benefits of proposed research outweigh risks to participants (Brody, 1998).

2.2.2. Free and Informed Consent

Informed consent is an essential condition of ethical research, and involves asking potential participants to consent to their participation after a detailed description of events that will occur in the course of the study (including description of possible risks and adverse events), and an opportunity to ask questions (Brody,

1998). The participation of persons under the age of 18 years may require the consent of a parent or guardian, along with the *assent* of the young person, though this will vary across jurisdictions. Any uncertainty about participation risks must be accurately communicated to potential participants along with close monitoring of adverse events that may occur, and remedial action where necessary.

All forms of consent must be given after participants are informed of what involvement in the research will require. Ideally, the consent process would include an independent witness to ensure the integrity of the process, and participants must be allowed to withdraw at any time (along with data collected). A participant's decision to withdraw must be respected and be free of consequences, such as incurred costs or refusal of future care (Brody, 1998).

The conditions under which persons are recruited into a study should be free from coercion or excessive inducement to participate (Brody, 1998). In recent years, it has become more common to reimburse study participants (i.e., via cash payment, vouchers, movie tickets, travel costs etc). However, cash payments may be interpreted by potential study participants as rewards for potential risks or harm. Under these circumstances, vouchers and money may serve as inducements for participation rather than as acceptable reimbursements for time and travel costs (Ashcroft, 2001).

2.2.3. Privacy and Confidentiality

Participant privacy is another ethical obligation that should be respected in any research. The privacy question refers to the extent to which a research study collects, uses or discloses identified or potentially identifiable information without individual consent. It encompasses 'confidentiality' (non disclosure of information and/or identity) and 'anonymity' (protection of participant identity). The basic accepted standard is that personal information must not be disclosed to any individual or group without participant consent, and participant identity should not be identifiable from the published results of the study (Brody, 1998).

2.2.4. Vulnerable Research Participants

Research involving persons who are cognitively or physically impaired or in a dependent relationship with investigators (e.g. as clients or students) requires special consideration (Brody, 1998). The most widely discussed issue is whether vulnerable persons are capable of providing informed consent in that they are able to: (1) understand the rationale for a research study; (2) understand what is required of them and why; and (3) provide free and informed consent to participate in the study (National Bioethics Advisory Commission, 1999). The scientific community hold differing views on the ability of vulnerable persons to give informed consent to research participation. A generally accepted model of practice is one that strives to protect special needs and minimize potential research harms (Brody, 1998).

3. ETHICAL ISSUES IN DRUG EPIDEMIOLOGICAL RESEARCH

3.1. Ethical Challenges in Drug Use Epidemiology

In most developed countries the institutional research ethics committees that oversee human research typically adhere to the broad ethical principles outlined above. However, questions exist about the applicability of such principles and standards to new and emerging fields of research. General ethical principles often fail to provide specific guidance in dealing with the complexities and ambiguities of ethical challenges that arise in everyday practice (Witkin, 2000). There are also concerns about how ethical standards and processes developed in one cultural context apply in settings where different research traditions may exist, or where morality and ethics are not institutionalized. We illustrate some of these concerns by considering some major unresolved ethical challenges in drug epidemiological research. Our aim is to highlight significant ethical challenges, rather than provide exhaustive analysis or solutions.

3.1.1. Free and Informed Consent

The adequacy of informed consent is commonly assessed in relation to questions about: the level of information provided to participants about research procedures, risks, benefits and safeguards; types of information delivery when considering literacy levels and preferred communication modes; opportunities for participants to voice concerns and ask questions; the extent to which consent is free from duress, undue influence or intimidation; and who has authority to provide consent.

Free and informed consent to participate in epidemiological research does not present any special problems for autonomous adults who can understand the nature of their participation and can freely decide to be involved or not. It presents more of an ethical issue for epidemiological studies of persons under the age of consent (Brody and Waldron, 2000), particularly when jurisdictional regulations differ. Obtaining consent can be cumbersome in school-based surveys of drug use (an efficient way of doing surveys of drug use). Typically low response rates and under-representation of minority groups has prompted researchers to use a method of "passive parental consent", in which a circular or letter informs parents that a survey is to be conducted and invites them to object to their child's participation. It is then assumed that the absence of parental objection means that the child can be included in school surveys. This approach requires further ethical justification and discussion.

3.1.1.a.   Impaired Consent. A special issue for epidemiological research on drug use and addiction is whether persons who are drug dependent have an impaired capacity to consent to participation in research. It has become an issue in the context of experimental and clinical research involving the administration of drugs of dependence (Charland, 2002; Cohen, 2002; College on Problems of Drug Dependence, 1995; Gorelick et al., 1999; Hall et al., 2003). Some (e.g. Charland, 2002; Cohen, 2002) have argued that the nature of addiction precludes an informed decision as to participation in experiments where a drug of dependence will be administered. It is uncertain how applicable these arguments are to epidemiological drug research, but the question of consent and impairment is clearly important.

Informed consent issues also arise for research participants who may be intoxicated, or who may have an acute drug induced psychiatric condition (Tarter et al., 1995). The College on Problems of Drug Dependence (1995) has suggested that informed consent should not be obtained when prospective participants are intoxicated, in withdrawal or cognitively impaired. However, it is unclear how a state of intoxication or impairment (of comprehension or performance) may be reliably determined. A key ethical consideration is the potential risks people may be exposed to because of their participation (e.g. increased intoxication and risk of overdose).

3.1.1.b.   Research Participant Payment. Participant payment in epidemiological research on drug use raises questions about voluntary consent. In Australia and the US for example, it has been common practice since the 1980s for researchers to pay illicit drug users for involvement in research (College on Problems of Drug Dependence, 1995). While the bioethics literature has explored research payment ethics (Grady, 2001; Macklin, 1981; McNeill, 1997; Wilkinson and Moore, 1997) it has not yet considered the special issues raised by paying drug users for research involvement. Critics of this practice are concerned that cash payments will serve as an inducement because they may be used to purchase drugs (Brody and Waldron, 2000). Non-cash payments (e.g. vouchers, prize draws, food and refreshments) have been suggested as more appropriate for this reason. Advocates of cash payments argue that payment for research participation is an ethical practice in that it reflects the ethical principles of respect and dignity (Grady, 2001; Ritter et al., 2003). Non-cash methods, they argue, reinforce negative drug user stereotypes and reflect a paternalistic view of the capacity and rights of users to make their own choices.

A key consideration is the potential for payments to increase risks to participants. Drug dependent persons may be vulnerable to coercion and inducement to participate in research when they are intoxicated or when they are experiencing acute withdrawal (College on Problems of Drug Dependence, 1995; Gorelick et al., 1999). In such cases, monetary payments may be seen as an inducement to participate because these enable the person to fund (even if only partially) the purchase of drugs to alleviate their withdrawal symptoms. Persons in this predicament may ignore any risks that participation entails that would in other circumstances discourage study entry.

To avoid these problems researchers may need to consider screening participants for withdrawal symptoms when assessing suitability and obtaining informed consent (College on Problems of Drug Dependence, 1995; Gorelick et al., 1999). Other strategies to consider include not advertising cash payments when recruiting participants or providing cash payment immediately after informed consent has been obtained and prior to interview/survey commencement (to minimise coercive impact of payment). This issue is controversial and remains unresolved in epidemiological drug research (Fry and Hall, 2003).

3.1.2.   Privacy, Confidentiality and Legal Hazard

Some types of drugs (e.g. cocaine and heroin) are illegal in any context and the use of some drugs is illegal in some age groups (e.g. alcohol use by persons under the minimum legal age). Drug use surveys may also ask about illegal and stigmatized acts, such as driving while intoxicated, selling illegal drugs or engaging in theft, fraud or violence to finance drug use. If law enforcement officials have access to such data and it can be linked to individuals then study participants could face criminal charges. In the US, researchers can obtain certificates of confidentiality in order to provide participants with an assurance that this will not happen. The situation in other countries is less clear (Fitzgerald and Hamilton, 1996; Loxley et al., 1996).

Participant privacy is a critical concern in drug epidemiological research. As stated previously, this encompasses protection of confidentiality and anonymity (i.e. non disclosure of information and/or identity without consent). Protecting the confidentiality of sensitive information collected through research is less of a problem when identifying information is not obtained (such as person's name or other unique identifiers) and anonymity thereby preserved. Ensuring confidentiality becomes more of an ethical issue in longitudinal studies where multiple contact details may be collected to allow individuals to be recontacted for follow-up interviews, months or even years later. Standard precautions are to store names and identifiers and the survey data separately and securely.

However, even when such protective measures are taken researchers in some countries may be compelled by courts to provide research records to law enforcement officials. Concerns around privacy also arise in the case of field research where face-to-face interviews may occur in public places such as the street, parks or cafes etc. In small communities this may create a potential risk to research participants, particularly if the investigator is a known drug researcher or if the interview is overheard.

Confidentiality is a potentially major ethical issue if biological samples (e.g. blood) are taken from a participant. DNA that can be extracted from such samples provides a unique identifier for all individuals (except identical twins). It could, if linked with questionnaire or interview data, permit individuals to be linked with self-reported illegal acts. The same issues are raised by the use of case registers and clinical databases, such as, treatment registers, or registers that linked treatment, arrest and other reporting of people who use drugs.

The implications for drug epidemiology of recent changes in a number of jurisdictions to health privacy and data protection legislation will require careful monitoring, and drug use epidemiologists should be aware of these (Lawlor and Stone, 2001). In jurisdictions where legislation requires identification and tracking of drug users, assurances of confidentiality cannot be given to participants. In such cases, researchers might seriously consider the option of not conducting the research.

3.1.3. Safety Issues

Illicit drug research often occurs in settings that may be dangerous for researchers and participants (Wright et al., 1998). In order to protect participant privacy, illicit drug users are often interviewed in settings out of the public gaze. Interviews may occur late at night, in the participants' residence, and other settings in which researcher safety cannot be guaranteed. Personal safety is an ethical issue to the extent that it is the responsibility of the researcher to ensure that their research, and contact with research participants and their communities, does not cause harm to research participants, researchers or community members. Safety protocols emerging for social science research (Craig et al., 2002) have potential for addressing safety issues in drug epidemiology.

3.2. Drug Epidemiological Research Challenges in Developing Countries

The ethical challenges posed by epidemiological research on drug use are amplified in comparative epidemiological studies of drug use across cultures (Council for International Organizations of Medical Sciences, 1991; Brody, 1998). This is particularly true in developing countries with little or no tradition of doing such research, and no institutional infrastructure for research ethics oversight that is standard in many developed societies. The application of broad biomedical ethical principles to this research may be a starting point but significant practical challenges exist that should also be addressed, such as developing local mechanisms for ethical decision-making and protection of research participants, (see Strauss et al., 2001).

One cannot assume that the rules of informed consent, privacy and confidentiality that have arisen out of debates on ethical principles in developed countries can be applied across all cultures and societies. For example, as a relatively recent development in research ethics, there are still many unanswered questions about the requirements of informed consent in these settings (Ijsselmuiden and Faden, 1999). Further, the relevance of issues such as participant vulnerability, awareness and expectations about rights, communication difficulties, documentation issues, literacy and the rules of obtaining consent in hierarchical societies are all still contested and deserve further attention (Sánchez et al., 2001).

4. CONCLUSIONS AND A WAY FORWARD

Consideration of ethical issues is crucial to biomedical, clinical and social research effort. While principles and guidelines that have emerged from biomedical ethics can assist in defining the ethical boundaries of most research, they provide limited guidance in relation to the day-to-day challenges that researchers encounter, particularly in speciality areas such as drug epidemiology. One way ahead for drug abuse epidemiology is to strive to apply the intent of ethical principles such as autonomy and beneficence, and the rules that derive from these to the analysis of specific cases through a process of open debate and discussion. This approach could inform discussions of ethical issues that arise in research in developing countries. We have explored these issues (including discussion of a hierarchy of ethical review options) more fully elsewhere (Fry and Hall, 2002; 2004).

Where to from here? Ethical analysis of epidemiological research on drug use is an under-developed field, even in developed societies with a tradition of drug research and ethical protection of human participants in medical research. Drug researchers must start to address the issues that are unique to drug abuse epidemiology in a more systematic way. The urgency of doing so is increased by recent efforts to expand epidemiological research on drug use to cultures and societies with little tradition of drug research, and often no experience in the ethical oversight of human medical research. Given the role of international organizations such as WHO and UNODC in sponsoring such research, these organizations may also consider facilitating future discussion and debate about ethical issues from which an applied ethical framework and resources for international drug abuse epidemiology may emerge.

ACKNOWLEDGEMENTS

Material for this chapter is adapted with permission from recent work supported by the United Nations Office on Drugs and Crime (Fry and Hall; 2002;

2004). Craig Fry is supported by funds from the 2003 Australian Museum and Australian Catholic University Eureka Prize for Research in Ethics.

REFERENCES

Agar, M. (1996). Recasting the 'ethno' in 'epidemiology'. *Medical Anthropology* 16, pp. 391–403.

Anthony, J. C., and Helzer, J. (1991). Syndromes of drug abuse and dependence. In: Robins L. N., and Regier, D. A. (Eds.), *Psychiatric Disorders in America.* Academic Press, New York, pp. 116–154.

Ashcroft, R. (2001). Selection of Human Research Subjects. In: Chadwick, R. (Ed.), *The Concise Encyclopedia of the Ethics of New Technologies*, Academic Press, New York, pp. 255–266.

Bachman, J. G., Wadsworth, K. N., O'Malley, P. M., Johnston, L. D., and Schulenberg, J. (1997). *Smoking, drinking and drug use in young adulthood: The impacts of new freedoms and responsibilities.* Lawrence Erlbaum: Mahwah NJ.

Beauchamp, T. L., and Childress, J. F. (2001). *Principles of Biomedical Ethics*, 5th ed. Oxford University Press, Oxford.

Brody, B. (1998). The Ethics of Biomedical Research: An International Perspective. Oxford University Press, New York.

Brody, J. L., and Waldron, H. B. (2000). Ethical issues in research on the treatment of adolescent substance abuse disorders. *Addictive Behaviors* 25, pp. 217–228.

Charland, L. C. (2002). Cynthia's dilemma: consenting to heroin prescription. *American Journal of Bioethics* 2, pp. 37–47.

Cohen, P. (2002). Untreated addiction imposes an ethical bar to recruiting addicts for non-therapeutic studies of addictive drugs. *Journal of Law, Medicine and Ethics* 30, pp. 73–81.

College on Problems of Drug Dependence (1995). Human subject issues in drug abuse research. *Drug and Alcohol Dependence* 37, pp. 167–175.

Coughlin, S. S. (2000). Ethics in epidemiology at the end of the 20th Century: Ethics, values and mission statements. *Epidemiologic Review* 22, pp. 169–175.

Council for International Organizations of Medical Sciences. (1991). International Guidelines for Ethical Review of Epidemiological Studies. Council for International Organizations of Medical Sciences (CIOMS), World Health Organization, Geneva.

Craig, G., Corden, A., and Thornton, P. (2002). Safety in social research. *Social Research Update* 29, pp. 1–6.

Ezzati, M., Lopez, A.D., Rodgers, A., Vander Hoorn, S., Murray, C.J. and the Comparative Risk Assessment Collaborating Group. (2002). Selected major risk factors and global and regional burden of disease. *Lancet* 28, pp. 1–14.

Fitzgerald, J., and Hamilton, M. (1996). Confidentiality, disseminated regulation and ethico-legal liabilities in research with hidden populations of illicit drug users. *Addiction* 92, pp. 1099–1107.

Fry, C. L., and Hall, W. (2002). An ethical framework for drug epidemiology: identifying the issues. *Bulletin on Narcotics* LIV(1–2), pp. 131–142.

Fry, C. L., and Hall, W. (2003). Key issues in determining the ethics of research subject payment: the special case of drug abuse epidemiology. *Australasian Epidemiologist* 10(1), pp. 41–47.

Fry, C. L., and Hall, W. (2004). Ethical challenges in drug epidemiology: Issues, principles and guidelines. Global Assessment Programme on Drug Abuse, Epidemiological Toolkit, Module VII. United Nations Office on Drugs and Crime, Vienna. http://www.unodc.org/unodc/en/drug_demand _gap_m-toolkit.html.

Gorelick, D., Pickens, R. W., and Benkovsky, F. O. (1999). Clinical research in substance abuse: human subjects issues. In Pincus, H. A., Lieberman, J. A. and Ferris, S. (Eds.), *Ethics in Psychiatric*

Research: A resource manual for human subjects protection. American Psychiatric Association, Washington, pp. 177–218.

Grady, C. (2001). Money for research participation: Does it jeopardize informed consent? *American Journal of Bioethics* 1, pp. 41–44.

Hall, W., Carter, L., and Morley, K. I. (2003). Addiction, neuroscience and ethics. *Addiction* 98, pp. 867–870.

Hser, Y. I., Hoffman, V., Grella, C. E., and Anglin, M. D. (2001). A 33-year follow-up of narcotic addicts. *Archives of General Psychiatry* 58, pp. 503–508.

Ijsselmuiden, C., and Faden, R. (1999). Research and informed consent in Africa: Another look. In: Mann, J. M., Gruskin, S., Grodin, M. A., and Annas, G. J. (Eds.), *Health and human rights: a reader.* Routledge, New York, pp. 363–372.

Jonsen, A. R. (1998). The Birth of Bioethics. Oxford University Press, New York, NY.

Kandel, D. B., and Chen, K. (2000). Types of marijuana users by longitudinal course. *Journal of Studies on Alcohol* 61, pp. 367–378.

LaFollete, H. (Ed.), (2001). *The Blackwell Guide to Ethical Theory.* Blackwell Publishers, Oxford.

Lawlor, D. A., and Stone, T. (2001). Public health and data protection: an inevitable collision or potential for a meeting of minds? *International Journal of Epidemiology* 30, pp. 1221–1225.

Loxley, W., Hawks, D., and Bevan, J. (1996). Protecting the interests of participants in research into illicit drug use: two case studies. *Addiction* 92, pp. 1081–1085.

Macklin, R. (1981). "Due" and "undue" inducements: On paying money to research subjects. *IRB: A Review of Human Subjects Research* 3, pp. 1–6.

Maher, L., Dixon, D., Lynskey, M., and Hall, W. (1998). Running the risks: heroin, health and harm in South-West Sydney. National Drug and Alcohol Research Centre, Sydney.

McNeill, P. (1997). Paying people to participate in research: Why not? *Bioethics* 11, pp. 390–396.

National Bioethics Advisory Commission (1999). Research Involving Persons with Mental Disorders That May Affect Decision Making Capacity. Rockville, Maryland.

Rachels, J. (1993). *The Elements of Moral Philosophy*, 2nd Ed. McGraw-Hill, New York.

Rawls, J. A. (1971). *Theory of Justice.* Oxford University Press, Oxford.

Ritter, A. J., Fry, C., and Swan, A. (2003). The ethics of reimbursing injecting drug users for public health research interviews: What price are we prepared to pay? *International Journal of Drug Policy* 14, pp. 1–3.

Roberts, M. J., and Reich, M. R. (2002). Ethical analysis in public health. *Lancet* 359, pp. 1055–1059.

Singer, P. (1993). *Practical Ethics*, 2nd Ed. Cambridge University Press, Cambridge.

Strauss, R. P., Sengupta, S., Quinn, S. C., Goeppinger, J., Spaulding, C., Kegeles, S. M., and Millett, G. (2001). The role of community advisory boards: Involving communities in the informed consent process. *American Journal of Public Health* 91(12), pp. 1938–1943.

Tarter, R. E., Mezzich, A. C., Hsieh, Y-C., and Parks, S. M. (1995). Cognitive capacity in female adolescent substance abusers. *Drug and Alcohol Dependence* 39, pp. 15–21.

Wilkinson, M., and Moore, A. (1997). Inducement in research. *Bioethics* 11, pp. 373–389.

Witkin, S. L. (2000). Ethics-R-Us. *Social Work* 45, pp. 197–200.

Wright, S., Klee, H., and Reid, P. (1998). Interviewing illicit drug users: observations from the field. *Addiction Research* 6, pp. 517–535.

C

Descriptive and Analytic Epidemiologic Studies

11

A Common Language for a Common Problem: The Developing Role of Drug Epidemiology in a Global Context

Paul Griffiths and Rebecca McKetin

PAUL GRIFFITHS • Coordinator of the Situation Analysis Programme, European Monitoring Centre for Drugs and Drug Addiction
REBECCA McKETIN • National Drug and Alcohol Research Centre, University of New South Wales Sydney

1. INTRODUCTION—TOWARDS A SHARED AGENDA

Each year, at the annual meeting of the United Nations' Commission on Narcotic Drugs (CND), a report is made on the global situation based on information submitted by member states following an agreed upon reporting protocol. Many aspects of the report are derived from data supplied by drug abuse epidemiology networks—or from drug information systems that include epidemiological elements. Not all countries supply information and for those that do the quality and comparability of what is supplied vary considerably. Nonetheless, this reporting process leads to a number of conclusions that would not have been evident even as short a time as a decade ago. The first of these is that the drug problem is now global in its nature. Many countries face a social phenomenon that, in some aspects at least, cuts across both national and cultural boundaries. For both developed and developing nations drug use is now recognized as an important issue for domestic as well as international policy. Historically this was not the case, the international debate more often reflected a polarization between a group of developing countries that produced drugs and a group of develop countries in which they were consumed.

The global nature of today's drug problem is clear from data reported by the United National Office on Drugs and Crime (UNODC), (World Drug Report 2004) based in part on the annual reporting exercise mentioned above (See Figure 1). In estimates of the annual consumption of cannabis, cocaine, and heroin it can be noted that in terms of the actual numbers of individual users the estimate for cocaine is highest for North America. Although in general estimates of rates of last year prevalence for the adult population of North America and Europe still tend to be somewhat higher than elsewhere in terms of the absolute number of individuals consuming illicit drugs, most are now living in the developing or transitional world. Furthermore, for a combination of reasons including globalization, urbanization, and demographic dynamics, drug use in the future is likely to become increasingly more common in developing countries. One simple example of this can be seen in an inspection of population age distribution data. In Figure 2, population pyramids are given for the United States (USA), Pakistan, Kazakhstan, and the United Kingdom (UK). It can be noted that the total number of

Region	Heroin Number in millions	Heroin % of adult population	Cocaine Number in millions	Cocaine % of adult population	Cannabis Number in millions	Cannabis % of adult population
Africa	0.8	0.17	0,94	0.21	34.60	7.7
Americas	1.42	0.26	8.70	1.57	34.9	6.3
N. America	1.24	0.45	6.38	2.30	28.5	10.3
S. America	0.18	0.07	2.32	0.84	6.5	2.4
Asia	4.13	0.17	0.15	0.01	44.7	1.9
Europe	2.75	0.51	3.34	0.62	28.8	5.3
W. Europe	1.27	0.41	3.11	1.01	20.4	6.7
E. Europe	1.48		0.23	0.10	8.4	3.6
Oceania	0.06	0.3	0.21	1.05	3.40	16.4
Global	9.16	0.23	13.34	0.34	146.3	3.7

Source: World Drug Report 2004 V1. Analysis, UNODC, 2004, United Nations Publication ISBN 92-1-148185-6

Figure 1. Global estimates of annual prevalence of Heroin, Cocaine and Cannabis.

those less than 15 years of age is similar in Pakistan and the USA, despite the fact that in overall population terms the USA is a far larger country. Drug problems tend to disproportionately impact on the urban young, and tend to be made more acute with the existence of other social difficulties and during periods of rapid social change. All these factors suggest that it is the developing, rather than the developed world that will disproportionately experience the drug epidemics of the future.

A caveat here is that this generalization ignores the fact that some developing countries had an historic concern about certain forms of domestic drug consumption. For example, a number of developing countries were active in ensuring the inclusion of cannabis in the drug control measures while the chewing of the psychoactive stimulant shoots of the Khat plant has long been a concern in Middle Eastern and some African countries and still effects migrant and refugee communities today (Griffiths et al., 1997). But historically, for most developing countries faced with a range of pressing health and social difficulties, drug use was rarely placed particularly high on their domestic agenda of concern. If it was recognized as an issue at all, the focus was more likely to be concern with the acculturated use of drugs by specific sub-cultural, indigenous, or ethnic sub-groups, rather than on the counter-culture of drug use by young people that characterized the drug problem from the 1960s onwards, in North America, Western Europe, and Australia. To a significant extent this now has changed and what was once characterized as the American disease (Musto, 1973) could perhaps now be better described as a global epidemic, or at least a social phenomenon to which few countries appear immune.

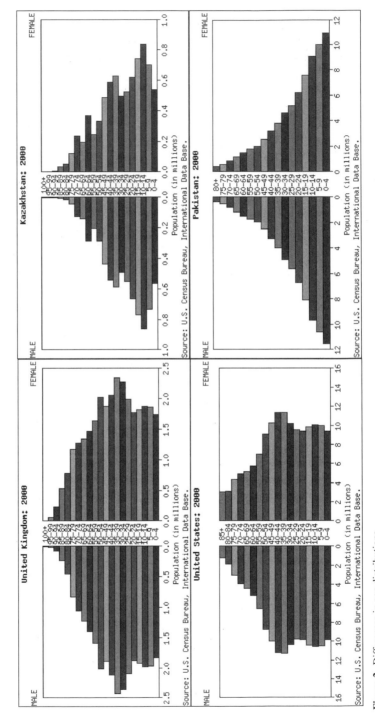

Figure 2. Differences in age distributions.

2.   BUILDING AN EVIDENCE-BASED RESPONSE—THE ROLE OF DRUG EPIDEMIOLOGY

This globalization of drug problems is reflected in the adoption of a set of common principles for a coordinated international community response. These principles can be summarized as: 1) support for the international drug control conventions, 2) commitment to a balanced approach that combines both demand and supply side elements, and 3) commitment to evidence-based policy making, reporting, and evaluation. The extent to which these internationally agreed-upon principles are reflected in the policies implemented by member states has varied. The drug control conventions are not without their critics and there are considerable differences evident in the way that they are interpreted within domestic policies and actions. While international agreement exists on the need for demand side measures, in practice for many countries they remain woefully underdeveloped or are even opposed. The support for evidence-based policy making while grounded on a sound understanding of the situation and using common and comparable methods is almost universally endorsed, but as some critical voices have noted (Fazey, 2002), information in this area is often highly politicized and often poorly reflects reality. In fact, the authoritative estimates given in Figure 1 are a little misleading as in some respects they are better described as "guesstimates" rather than as empirically based statistics. Nonetheless they are illustrative of a sincere attempt to quantify the drug situation even if the commitments to this endeavor of individual governments may vary. The result of this process has been that the necessary political support has been provided for the establishment and development of drug epidemiological systems around the world. Such support has sometimes faltered and at the international level it has often been a case of two-steps forward followed by one step back. However, despite this tentative movement, progress has been made and some commonalities are observable in both the activities undertaken and the structures that have been developed to support them.

3.   DRUG CONTROL AND PUBLIC HEALTH: TWIN ENGINES FOR THE DEVELOPMENT OF DRUG EPIDEMIOLOGICAL ACTIVITIES

Many of today's activities with respect to the epidemiology of drug use have a strong public health perspective. However, historically an equally important, and arguably at times the predominant engine behind the development of information systems on drug use, has been the various national and international acts and agreements designed to prohibit the consumption of psychoactive substances. Indeed it was the need to monitor the impact of drug control measures in the USA that first generated the interest for epidemiological inquiry to establish the 'true' scale of the problem (Musto and Sloboda, 2003).

Drug control policies had developed in America following concern around the health impact of the use of cocaine and opium products and a growing public recognition of the dangers of addiction and 'moral deterioration' that these products could cause. Despite some opposition from the pharmaceutical industry, the Harrison Act of 1914 placed control on the distribution of narcotics (Musto, 1973). International control policies were also developing at this time with the first international treaty to control trafficking in opiates and cocaine being formulated in The Hague in 1912. Today drug control is regulated at the global level by series of United Nations conventions and within these are obligations for assessment and reporting that provide a concrete rationale for drug epidemiological activities.

3.1. International Conventions on Narcotics Control and Global Reporting Obligations

International control of narcotic substances was first implemented through the United Nations in 1961, under the Single Convention on Narcotic Drugs (United Nations, 1961), this convention was later amended in 1971 to include psychotropic substances (e.g., amphetamine-type stimulants), and later fortified in 1988 (Bayer and Ghodse, 1999; United Nations, 1961; 1971; 1981; 1991; 1993) to include controls on precursor chemicals for synthetic drugs.

The international conventions have generated awareness on the need to understand the drug problem and have stimulated a more concerted effort to monitor trends in drug use in order to facilitate more effective drug control strategies. Although activities are driven in part by the need to monitor progress toward meeting obligations under drug control conventions, an increasingly important argument for many member states has been the need to understand and circumvent public health consequences of drug use, particularly those related to infectious diseases. These twin objectives have since been united in the 1998, UNGASS—Political Declaration of United Nations Member States (United Nations 1998) stating that drug control should reflect a balanced approach between controlling drug supply and reducing demand for illicit drugs. This declaration also recommended that responses to the drug situation be based on "*a regular assessment of the nature and magnitude of drug use and abuse and drug-related problems in the population*" and set targets for member states to work towards.

Reporting obligations to the United Nations conventions are implemented through the Annual Reports Questionnaire (ARQ) which contains three parts. Part I addresses information on the adherence to the conventions and legal measures; Part II describes the extent and nature of the problem, and Part III collects information on interdiction measures (such as drug seizures). Part II can be thought of as basically containing epidemiological data on drug use and was recently re-vised to reflect a consensus on what constituted good practice in reporting this kind of information at a global level. A second global instrument is the Biennial Reports Questionnaire used to collect information relevant to the assessment of progress made in respect of the UNGASS targets.

3.2. Elements of Drug Monitoring—Indicators and Methods

As the initial development of drug abuse epidemiology was driven by the need to monitor the impact of control activities, prevalence was clearly a key question. Indeed the drug debate has always been characterized by arguments about the scale of the problem. In the USA inflated estimates of the number of drug abusers were made by proponents of the Harrison Act to circumvent amendments to the legis-lation designed to allow opioid maintenance therapy. Similarly, evidence exists to suggest that later American estimates appear to reflect political concerns or needs rather than directly representing the scale of the problem. In response to this prob-lem, and following the dramatic rise in drug use in the 1960s, the Comprehensive Drug Abuse and Control Act of 1970 included the commissioning of an informed and independent evaluation of the drug problem through the 'National Commis-sion on Marihuana and Drug Abuse'. The lack of reliable existing estimates of drug use lead to the development of population surveys to monitor drug use, the first of these occurring in 1974, closely followed by comparable surveys among school students in 1975 (Musto and Sloboda, 2002). Repeating these surveys on a periodic basis allowed monitoring of the prevalence of drug use among the general population and among school students and represented the first use of large-scale population surveys to monitor the drug situation. Thirty years on these surveys have provided a valuable indication of shifts in the number of people using drugs over time, and have also been used to estimate trends in the number of new drugs. General population surveys of drug use are now an internationally recognized tool for assessing drug use but credible national level exercises of this sort remain re-stricted, with notable exceptions, to the developed world. The limitation of the use of surveys is in part because they are expensive, methodologically demanding, and often perform poorly in respect to the assessment of levels of chronic drug use. Also for countries with poor instructional record keeping and/or public distrust of the authorities, they are difficult to do at all. Although some of these limitations also apply to school surveys, this method has been more widely adopted interna-tionally. Today school survey data provide the most comprehensive global data set for looking at patterns of drug use across countries and regions. The European School Project on Alcohol and Drugs (ESPAD) now embraces over 30 countries (Hibell et al., 1999), the Organization of American States (OAS/CICAD) has been supporting school survey work across the Americas and the Caribbean. School surveys are also being administered in an increasing number of Asian and African countries, and are found in virtually all developed countries (Douglas and Hillebrand, 2003).

In addition to the use of population surveys a range of other methodological approaches has developed to understand the nature and scale of illicit drug use. These include sociological surveys of drug-using populations, clinical/psychiatric research on treatment populations or other institutional populations, criminological studies on incarcerated drug users, and the use of law enforcement data. Many of these methods are discussed elsewhere in this book. In terms of the international development of epidemiological monitoring systems it is worth making a special note of the importance of treatment-based monitoring systems which form the mainstay of many contemporary drug information systems. The success of treatment reporting as a data collection option rests on a number of factors including the fact that this is a relatively easy and low cost method for reporting on the most chronic forms of drug problems, appropriate to any country that has some form of drug treatment, and that the relevance of this kind of information is easily understood by clinicians, policy makers and the general public.

Early treatment data collection systems developed in the late 1960s to early 1970s notably including the *Home Office Addict Notification Index* in the United Kingdom (Mott, 1994), where doctors reported on the number of patients presenting with opiate drug problems. Registers of drug-related presentations to mental health facilities are also common such as in Indonesia and Japan as is the collection of admission and discharge data from federally funded treatment programs such as in the United States of America (for a review see Stauffacher, 2002). Contemporary development of treatment demand data has seen improvements in comparability and coverage. In Europe the standardized collection of treatment demands has been a key part of the development of a European reporting system. From 1991, the Pompidou Group of the Council of Europe began developing and piloting a standardized protocol for collecting core items of treatment data which could be used by professionals and researchers across Europe. This Treatment Demand Protocol was finalized in 1994. Since 2000 treatment demand data have been collected across the European Union and in many Central and Eastern European countries under the joint protocol of the Pompidou Group and the European Monitoring Centre for Drugs and Drug Addiction (EMCDDA). Comparable collections of treatment data across Europe has provided an indicator of regional trends in treatment demand and has also allowed for cross-country comparisons. In Figure 3 examples of data from treatment reporting systems can be found. This information facilitates the understanding of the differing nature of the drug problem between and across different countries and regions; for example the growing opiate problem in Central Asia and the importance of amphetamine related problems in Scandinavian countries.

In some countries, treatment demand data are combined with information on drug users from other sources, notably arrest data, to develop a register of all

A). Main drug problem among treatment clients by country, 2001 (Source EMCDDA 2003)

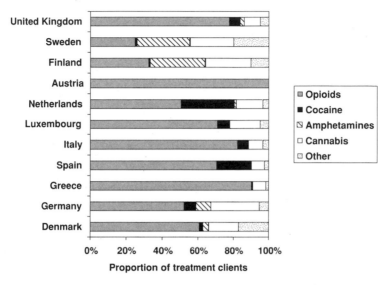

B). Central Asian Republics: Drug Users Registered per 100,000 population (cumulative). (Source UNODP, Niaz 2001)

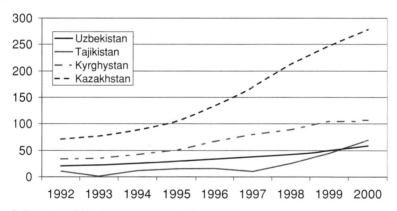

Figure 3. Examples of data from treatment reporting systems.

'known' drug users. It is important to note that such systems only represent drug users who come into contact with participating agencies, and therefore cannot provide incidence or prevalence data but, as with other routine indicators, these registries can provide information on drug trends. A good example of such a registry is the Central Registry of Drug Abuse in the special administrative region of

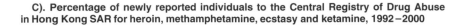

C). Percentage of newly reported individuals to the Central Registry of Drug Abuse in Hong Kong SAR for heroin, methamphetamine, ecstasy and ketamine, 1992–2000

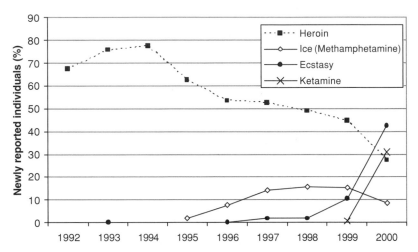

Figure 3. *Continued.*

Hong Kong. This system has been maintaining information reported from treatment, law enforcement, and welfare agencies since 1976 (Stauffacher, 2002). Data from this registry have been important in documenting the rise in synthetic drugs (i.e., ecstasy, methamphetamine and ketamine) over the past decade, which in many nearby countries can only be noted from anecdotal evidence (UNODC, 2004).

In addition to treatment and law enforcement data, a range of other drug-related routine data sources have been used to monitor the drug situation, alongside surveys and other more specialized research efforts. Some of these data were established as early warning systems to detect emergent drug trends. For example the use of drug mentions among emergency attendances in cities throughout the United States (DAWN) to detect new trends was established in the 1970s and is still operating today. Law enforcement data on drug offences and drug seizures were another frequently used information source to track trends in drug use, and was particularly useful in settings where the opportunity to use health-related data on drug use was limited. In Japan, for example, arrest data date back to 1970 and can be used in conjunction with data from psychiatric registers to monitor trends in methamphetamine use, the country's dominant drug problem (UNODC, 2004). These types of routine data sources provide information on trends that could complement information from population surveys, the findings of sociological research on drug use patterns and other qualitative and clinical research.

3.3.   Networks, Multi-Indicator Models and Drug Information Systems

It became increasingly recognized that a single data source alone does not sufficiently capture the dynamic nature of drug use trends and often only provides a partial picture of the overall drug situation (Hartnoll, 2003). A strong argument therefore existed for a more integrated approach that combined data from different sources to gain a holistic view of the overall drug situation. This has prompted the creation of expert networks that have to a large extent shaped the international development of drug epidemiological systems. As well as having the benefit of bringing together experts with data from a range of sources, networking provides opportunities to gather information from different geographical areas thus contributing to a better national, regional, or even global picture.

An influential example of this multi-disciplinary approach is the Community Epidemiology Working Group in the United States of America (CEWG) (Sloboda and Kozel, 2003) that was established in the 1970s and was followed some time later by the Epidemiological network of the Pompidou Group (PG) of the Council of Europe, established in 1982 (Bless, 2003). Although these systems evolved separately, with the initial work of the PG influenced by European researchers attending CEWG meetings, there are strong parallels in their structure. Both systems are based on a network of interested experts and are relatively independent of local authorities and government structures. Both incorporate epidemiological data from sources thought to be core to monitoring drug trends (e.g., treatment data, arrest data). And finally, both incorporate expert opinion from people familiar with the local drug situation who are involved with obtaining the epidemiological data for inclusion in monitoring. Local knowledge facilitated accurate interpretation of indicator data by providing information on factors that influence the data (e.g., changes in provision of drug treatment) and also explained typical patterns of drug use and the situations in which drug use occurred, thereby providing an interpretive context for trend data.

During the 1970s systems to monitor drugs were predominantly the domain of Western Europe and North America. However, the following decades saw drug use becoming a global issue marked by the spread of injecting drug use to affect over 130 countries worldwide (Dehne et al., 2002). The spread of injecting drug use to become a worldwide epidemic together with the growing global epidemic of the Human Immunodeficiency Virus (HIV) presented a potentially devastating public health problem that required urgent preventative action. Prevention strategies necessarily required an understanding of where injecting drug use was prevalent, how large was the potential pool of injectors who might become infected with the virus, the extent of HIV infection among injecting drug users, and an understanding of related risk factors. These information needs were associated with the growth of several drug research methodologies, including sociological and ethnographic research on 'hidden' populations of drug users to understand HIV risk behavior, epidemiological methods to monitor the prevalence and incidence of blood borne viruses among injecting drug use, and indirect prevalence estimation methods to estimate the size of injecting drug use populations.

3.4. HIV and the Need for Information for Action—The Role of Rapid Assessment

The urgency of responding to the problem of injecting drug use in resource-poor settings was a key factor in the development of the 'rapid assessment' approach in the 1990s. The principle behind rapid assessment techniques was to draw from a variety of social science methodologies to undertake a quick and pragmatic assessment of the drug situation and risk factors for transmission of HIV. Information from the rapid assessment could then be used to design appropriate interventions to prevent the spread of HIV among the injecting population. Most rapid assessment studies rely on a mixture of survey methods and ethnographic research and the collection of biological data (i.e., HIV status) where relevant. Rapid assessment studies have now been undertaken in at least 70 countries (Fitch et al., 2002) and the methodology has been popularized to serve a broad range of objectives and encompass an array of social science methods.

4. GLOBAL PLAYERS—INTERNATIONAL ORGANIZATIONS, REGIONAL COOPERATION INITIATIVES AND TECHNICAL NETWORKS

Today, greater international trade, communication, and migration means patterns of drug use can rapidly transcend national borders and countries' drug problems can impact regional economic and political stability. In this context the monitoring of regional drug trends has become a more important policy issue. This has meant in practice that there has been a gradual movement away from loosely structured networks of experts to more institutional bodies that develop regional information systems. That said, the global picture remains somewhat heterogeneous and at regional levels, expert technical networks sometimes exist in tandem with more institutional bodies or have become integrated with them.

Of the main international bodies supporting drug epidemiological work, the three most prominent are The World Health Organization (WHO), that recently published an excellent drug epidemiological sourcebook (WHO 2000), UNAIDS with interests mainly focused on drug injecting, and UNODC that developed the Global Assessment Programme (GAP) supporting the development of regional epidemiological systems using an epidemiological toolkit specifically designed for data collection in developing countries (http://www.unodc.org/unodc/en/drug_demand_gap_m-toolkit.html).

At the regional level a number of key bodies can be identified. In the Americas a number of strong nation systems work with the OAS evaluation mechanism that includes a number of epidemiological elements (although the specific case of USA is somewhat different because of the considerable extent of national activities). Currently plans also exist for a monitoring center to be established for the Southern and Central American Countries. In Europe, the Pompidou Group remains active in methodological development but routine monitoring is now the responsibility of the European Monitoring Centre on Drugs and Drug Addiction (EMCDDA). This agency, based in Lisbon, Portugal, is one of the decentralized technical agencies of the European Commission. Around thirty countries are participating in the EMCDDA reporting system (European Union member states, applicant countries, and those joining by special arrangement). In Africa, a strong national system in South Africa has been used as a model for a regional initiative (Parry et al., 2003) and limited activities exist elsewhere with UNODCP supported networks in Central and Northern regions. The long established Asian multi-city study is still active but has been joined by a number of new regional activities, prompted in part by the methamphetamine epidemic affecting this area.

4.1.   Guiding Principles of Data Collection—The Lisbon Consensus*

Integral to efforts to improve international data on drug consumption is the harmonization of data collection methods and activities. An important first step in achieving this objective was taken in January 2000 with a joint meeting of representatives from international bodies, regional drug information networks, and other relevant technical experts. Particular consideration was given by the international expert panel to the development of a set of core epidemiological demand indicators for assessing drug consumption at a global level. A consensus statement was issued and subsequently positively noted by the Commission on Narcotics Drugs (United Nations, 2000). This consensus statement identified a number of core indicators of drug demand. These were: drug consumption among the general population, drug consumption among the youth population, high-risk drug abuse, service utilization for drug problems, drug related morbidity, and drug related mortality. These indicators were chosen as they address areas in which routine data collection was considered possible at least for some countries although they are not intended to represent a comprehensive information base required to address all needs at a regional or national level.

In addition to consensus on the core indicators of drug consumption, there was agreement on the principles that were needed to support data collection activities.

* This section of this paper is an abridged version of the paper 'Developing a global perspective on drug consumption patterns and trends—the challenge for drug epidemiology—*Bulletin on Narcotics*, 55(1 and 2), pp. 83–94.

The following 10 broad principles were noted: 1) data should be timely and relevant to the needs of policy makers and service providers, 2) while not sufficient in themselves for a comprehensive understanding of patterns of drug consumption, efforts to improve the comparability and quality of data at the international level should focus on a limited number of indicators and a manageable priority core data set, 3) simple indicators of drug consumption must be subject to appropriate analysis before strategic conclusions can be drawn using both qualitative and quantitative research and with broader information on context, 4) multi-method and multi-source approaches are of particular benefit in the collection and analysis of data on drug consumption and its consequences, 5) data should be collected in accordance with sound scientific methodological principles to ensure reliability and validity, 6) methods need to be adaptable and sensitive to the different cultures and contexts in which they are to be employed, 7) data collection, analysis, and reporting should be as consistent and comparable as possible in order to facilitate meaningful discussions of changes, similarities and differences in the drug phenomenon, 8) methods and sources of information should be clearly stated and open to review, 9) data collection and reporting should be in accordance with recognized standards of research ethics, and 10) data collection should be feasible and cost-effective in the terms of the national context where it occurs.

The consensus statement also noted that the identification of good methods alone is not sufficient for improving data collection capacity as it is also necessary to develop appropriate networks and organizational structures to provide the infrastructure necessary to support data collection. There is a need for improved capacity to analyze and interpret information on drug consumption applying good methods, well-trained and competent researchers, and appropriate resources. This in turn requires training and technical support, ongoing political support, and long-term and stable investment in this area to ensure sustainability and success of data collection systems. While expenditure on data collection has to be cost effective given the resources available within a country, the investment in data collection activities must be seen as both necessary and resource efficient in that it improves the development, targeting, and evaluation of other demand reduction investments.

5.   CONCLUDING REMARKS

At the international level, drug policy remains a politically charged issue and one that is entwined with sensitive policy issues including money laundering, crime, terrorism, and security. Member states have their own internal and external political agendas and considerable debate exists between those who call for either the liberalization of policy options and those who see a need for caution and renewed efforts at control. Against this complex realpolitk agenda stands the simple tenet that drug policies, whatever their nature, should be evidence-based. For drug epidemiologists working at the international level this means that they must strive to maintain sound scientific principles, knowing that the data they produce will be interpreted without regard to the careful caveats they put on it, and knowing that they will be criticized by those who feel that the available evidence does not support their chosen view. It has been argued that these political tensions mean that data produced at the international level is so tainted that it is of little worth. Certainly there are examples of the misuse of information and of the misinterpretation of data, without regard to scientific principles (Rossi, 2002). Nonetheless, there has been much progress toward improving data collection not only in terms of the coverage of data collection activities but also in terms of the quality of data collected and its utility in formulating policy. The use of drug information networks has played a key role in this developmental process, providing an opportunity for dialogue across different sectors of the community and between different countries and regions. Progress toward improving coverage of specific core indicators of drug use has been achieved in developing regions through the adaptation of cost-effective data collection methods. In this regard, epidemiological networks have been crucial in encouraging the systematic collection and interpretation of data from drug treatment services and other data on drug-related events. Challenges to further improve the coverage of these data collection activities and to expand drug information systems to foster the development of drug-related data collection activities remain. In the quicksand of policy debate and opinion the role of drug abuse epidemiologists can only be to provide a bedrock understanding of what is known and what is not known about the drug situation. It is the responsibility of others to ensure that this translates into better policies and actions.

REFERENCES

Bayer, I. and Ghodse, H. (1999). Evolution of international drug control, 1945–1995. *Bulletin on Narcotics*, 51(1 and 2), pp. 1–17.
Bless, R. (2003). Experiences of the multi-city network of the Pompidou Group, 1983–2002. In *Bulletin on Narcotics, vol. 55, no 1 and 2*. United Nations World Drug Report 2004, New York and United Nations Office on Drugs and Crime, United Nations Publications, Vienna, Austria, pp. 31–40.
Dehne, K.L., Adelekan, M., Chatterjee, A., and Weiler, G. (2002). The need for a global understanding of epidemiological data to inform human immunodeficiency virus (HIV) prevention among injecting drug users. *Bulletin on Narcotics* 54(1 and 2), pp. 117–142.
Douglas, K.G. and Hillebrand, J. (2003). The Caribbean epidemiological network: the complexities of developing a regional perspective. *Bulletin on Narcotics* 55(1 and 2), pp. 73–82.
Fazey, C. (2002). Commentary: estimating the world illicit drug situation—reality and the seven deadly political sins. *Drugs: Education, Prevention and Policy* 9(1), Taylor & Francis, London, pp. 95–103.
Fitch, C., Rhodes, T., Hope, V., Stimson, G.V., and Renton, A. (2002). The role of rapid assessment methods in drug use epidemiology. *Bulletin on Narcotics* 54(1 and 2), pp. 61–72.
Griffiths, P. Gossop M., Wickenden, S., Dunworth, K., Harris, K., and Lloyd C. (1997). A transcultural pattern of drug use: qat (khat) in the UK. *British Journal of Psychiatry 170*, pp. 281–284.

Hartnoll, R. (2003). Drug epidemiology in the European institutions: historical background and key indicators. *Bulletin on Narcotics* 55(1 and 2), pp. 53–72.

Hibell, B., Andersson, B., Ahlstrom, S., Balakireva, O., Bjarnasson, T., Kokkavi, A., and Morgan M. (1999). *The 1999 ESPAD report—Alcohol and other drugs in 30 European Countries.* The Swedish Council for information on Alcohol and Other Drugs (CAN) and The Pompidou Group of the Council of Europe.

Mott, J. (1994). Notification and the Home Office. In: Strang, J. and Gossop, M. (Eds.), *Heroin Addiction and Drug Policy: the British System,* Oxford, Oxford University Press, Chapter 21.

Musto, D. (1973). *The American Disease: Origins of Narcotic Control.* Yale University Press, New Haven and London.

Musto D.F. and Sloboda Z. (2003). The influence of epidemiology on drug control policy. *Bulletin on Narcotics,* 55(1 and 2), pp. 9–22.

Niaz, K. (2002). *Illicit Drug Use Trends in Central Asia.* Global Workshop on Drug Information Systems: Activities, Methods and Future Opportunities. December 3–5, 2001. Vienna International Centre, Austria. United Nations, Vienna.

Parry, C.D.H., Plüddemann, A., and Strijdom J. (2003). Developing the Southern African Development Community Epidemiology Network on Drug Use: methods and issues. *Bulletin on Narcotics* 55(1 and 2). pp. 83–94.

Rossi, C. (2002). Review essay: A critical reading of the World Drug Report 2000. *International Journal of Drug Policy* 13, pp. 221–231.

Sloboda, Z. and Kozel, N.J. (2003). Understanding drug trends in the United States of America: the role of the Community Epidemiology Work Group as part of a comprehensive drug information system. *Bulletin on Narcotics* 55(1 and 2), pp. 41–52.

Stauffacher, M. (2002). Drug treatment data as an epidemiological indicator: methodological considerations and improved analyses. *Bulletin on Narcotics* 54(1 and 2), pp. 73–85.

United Nations. (1961). *Single Convention on Narcotic Drugs, 1961, As Amended by the 1972 Protocol Amending the Single Convention on Narcotic Drugs, 1961.* http://www.unodc.org/pdf/convention_1961_en.pdf.

United Nations. (1971). *Convention on Psychotropic Substances, 1971.* http://www.unodc.org/pdf/convention_1971_en.pdf.

United Nations. (1988). *Convention against the Illicit Traffic in Narcotic Drugs and Psychotropic Substances, 1988.* http://www.unodc.org/pdf/convention_1988_en.pdf.

United Nations. (1991). United Nations *Convention against illicit traffic in narcotic drugs and psychotropic substances, 1988.* United Nations, New York.

United Nations. (1993). *Single convention on narcotic drugs, 1961: as amended by the 1972 Protocol Amending the Single Convention on Narcotic Drugs, 1961,* United Nations, New York.

United Nations, (1998). *Proceedings United Nations 20th Special Session. Political Declaration and Guiding Principles of Drug Demand Reduction,* United Nations, New York.

United Nations. 3 March 2000. *Drug Information Systems: Principles, Structures and Indicators.* (E/CN.7/CRP3).

United Nations Office on Drugs and Crime. (2004). *Amphetamine-type stimulant use in East Asia and the Pacific.* UNODC Regional Centre for East Asia and the Pacific, Bangkok.

World Health Organization. (2000). *Guide to drug abuse epidemiology,* Geneva, World Health Organization Geneva.

12

Longitudinal Studies of Drug Use and Abuse

Thomas A. Wills, Carmella Walker, and Jody A. Resko

THOMAS A. WILLS, CARMELLA WALKER, AND JODY A. RESKO • Albert Einstein College of Medicine

1.   LONGITUDINAL STUDIES OF DRUG USE AND ABUSE

In this chapter we discuss longitudinal studies investigating variables related to substance use and abuse. The emphasis is on research with general-population samples that has assessed participants at relatively early ages and followed them over time to examine how predictor variables are related to outcomes at later ages. Excluded are studies of persons already showing drug abuse (see Chapter 3), research with clinical samples of adolescents, and studies that started in late adolescence, when most persons who are going to use substances have already done so. The outcomes include intensity of tobacco, alcohol, and marijuana use; continuous measures of substance-related problems; or diagnostic assessments such as alcohol abuse. Such studies clarify questions about predictive relations through establishing variables that are true antecedents of drug use. They also help clarify the understanding of drug abuse through indicating risk factors and protective factors, conceptualized as distinct domains because risk and protection indices are not highly correlated (Newcomb and Felix-Ortiz, 1992).

Data on how the prevalence of substance use varies with age in general populations are available from several sources including Monitoring the Future and the National Household Survey on Drug Abuse (e.g., Johnston et al., 2000). Such studies show that substance use before the age of 11 years is infrequent but between the ages of 12 and 18 years, rates of substance use increase to a level where a substantial part of the population has used cigarettes or alcohol, and a smaller but not insignificant proportion shows problem use (e.g., Harrison et al., 1998). This makes longitudinal research during this period useful for helping to inform theory about the origins of substance abuse.

A general model of liability to substance abuse is presented in Figure 1. Factors operating in childhood may predispose to early onset of drug use, around 12 years of age. For a subgroup of teens, substance use onset is followed by escalation in the frequency and intensity of use (Wills et al., 1996). A high level of use can then lead to development of abuse or dependence for some persons, either in adolescence or at later ages (e.g., Wills et al., 2002). Risk factors increase liability for substance abuse through promoting early and/or escalated use, while protective factors reduce the likelihood of onset and escalation. Other factors may operate as direct effects (not through level of use), so individuals could be more or less vulnerable to problem use at a given level of substance use. This model, recognizing both indirect effects of predictors through promoting higher levels of use, and direct effects to abuse, underlies much of the research discussed in this chapter.

2.   STUDIES WITH BROAD-BASED MODELS

Here we discuss early studies that continue to influence current research. Sample sizes were in the range from 1,000 to 2,000 participants. These studies

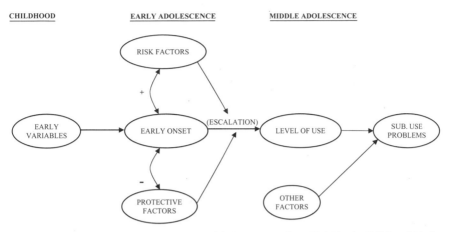

Figure 1. Model for Longitudinal Prediction of Substance Use from Variables in Childhood, Early Adolescence, Middle Adolescence and Late Adolescence/Early Adulthood. (Curved double-headed arrows indicate concurrent effects; straight single-headed arrows indicate cross-time effects. Paths are assumed to have positive coefficient unless otherwise noted;—indicates inverse coefficient.)

tested broad-based models assuming that drug abuse is linked to some combination of individual, family, and peer factors.

2.1. Social Adaptation Approach

In the Woodlawn Project, a large sample of mostly African-American children was assessed at 6 years of age; teacher and maternal reports were obtained about children's symptomatology and academic readiness. The sample was followed into adolescence (16 years of age) and adulthood (32 years of age). In adolescence, substance use was found to be elevated among males who had been rated in first grade as aggressive, while ratings of shyness were inversely related to substance use; among females, only ratings of psychological distress in first grade predicted adolescent substance use (Kellam et al., 1982). In adulthood, shyness in childhood and school bonding during adolescence predicted less marijuana use among women; among men, the combination of aggression and shyness in childhood predicted current marijuana and cocaine use (Ensminger et al., 2002). Early ratings of underachievement were related to alcohol abuse and dependence in adulthood, while adolescent data indicating that parents helped with homework and set clear rules for school behavior were indicated as protective factors.

2.2. Epidemiologic Approach

Epidemiologic research by Kandel and colleagues (1978) was based on a large sample of high school students in New York State and emphasized social predictors of substance use. Transitions to illicit drug use were predicted by factors such as parental substance use and lack of closeness to parents; delinquency; availability of drugs; and peer substance use. Follow-ups through age 34–35 years have delineated the natural history of drug use (e.g., Kandel et al., 1992); for example, alcohol use tended to peak around age 18 whereas cocaine use peaked in the mid-20s (Chen and Kandel, 1995). Several papers from this study have noted the adverse consequences of drug involvement in adolescence (e.g., Kandel et al., 1986).

2.3. Problem Behavior Approach

Problem behavior theory (Jessor and Jessor, 1977) locates the predisposing factors for substance use in rejection of conventional values and adoption of a deviance-prone attitudinal structure (e.g., tolerance for deviant behaviors such as stealing and fighting). School-based studies following middle-school students and college students showed prevalence (and onset) of problem drinking and marijuana use related to variables such as attending church infrequently, having low grades, being loosely attached to parents, having relative tolerance for deviance, and affiliating with deviant peers such as drinkers and marijuana users; correlations were also found among indices of heavy drinking, marijuana use, and sexual behavior (e.g., Donovan and Jessor, 1985). There was a decline in rates of substance use after adolescence, but a subgroup of persons showed sustained high levels of use from late adolescence to young adulthood (Donovan et al., 1991; Bachman et al., 2002). Recently problem behavior theory has been extended to prediction of other health behaviors (e.g., Jessor et al., 1998).

2.4. Personality Approach

In a 6-wave study by Newcomb, Bentler, and colleagues, participants were surveyed in middle schools (7th–9th grades) and then followed through high school and into young adulthood. This project tested a model emphasizing personality and attitudinal unconventionality as predictors and considering various consequences of use including academic and vocational adjustment (Newcomb and Bentler, 1988a). Problematic drug use (e.g., daily marijuana use) showed an almost linear relation to a 10-item risk-factor composite including variables such as social nonconformity, early alcohol use, low self-esteem, and poor relationship with parents (Newcomb et al., 1986). The investigators considered ethnic differences, finding African-American adolescents to have the lowest rates of substance use, and used structural equation modeling to determine predictors and consequences of substance use involvement. Analyses showed substance use positively related to factors such as life stress (Newcomb and Harlow, 1986) and inversely related to parental emotional support (Newcomb and Bentler, 1988b); problem outcomes (e.g., drunk driving) were related to coping motives for drug use (Newcomb et al., 1988). This study found many adverse consequences of adolescent substance use, with control for initial use; these included mental health problems, physical health problems, and relationship problems in adulthood (Newcomb and Bentler, 1988a,b).

2.5. Psychopathology Approach

Research by Brook and colleagues (1995) was based on a community sample of families in upstate New York, originally assessed when child participants were 1–10 years of age (mean age 5.6 years) and followed with assessments in early adolescence, late adolescence, and early adulthood (mean ages 22 and 27 years). This research used a model focused on individual psychopathology and family factors as predictors of drug abuse. Analyses for drug use in young adulthood showed childhood measures of aggression and temper tantrums to be significant predictors over a 20-year time span; adolescent measures of impulsivity and sensation seeking were risk factors for subsequent drug use, while adolescent measures of good self-control and moral beliefs were protective. This study also found heavy drug use in adolescence was related to adverse outcomes at later ages (e.g., Brook et al., 1999, 2002).

3. RECENT THEORY-TESTING STUDIES

During the past 10 years, studies with various designs have tested focused theoretical models about the origins of liability to substance abuse. Here we discuss representative studies that have tested questions such as the role of temperament and self-control factors, social influences, and family history of substance abuse.

3.1. Temperament and Self-Control Models

Studies influenced by temperament theory (Rothbart and Ahadi, 1994) have tested early-developing dispositional characteristics as predictors of substance use. An investigation with a sample of Finnish children initially assessed at 8–9 years of age (Pulkkinen and Pitkänen, 1994) found problem drinking in adulthood predicted by early ratings of poor concentration ability, high aggressiveness and low prosociality, and poor school performance. Mâsse and Tremblay (1997) used teacher ratings of children assessed at ages 6 and 10 years, subsequently coded for dimensions from Cloninger's (1987) personality theory, and found that the characteristics of novelty seeking and harm avoidance were significant predictors for drunkenness, cigarette smoking, and other drug use during adolescence. A study of a birth cohort in New Zealand (Caspi et al., 1996) obtained temperament assessments at 3 years of age and followed participants with periodic assessments including diagnostic interviews at age 21 years. A group characterized as "Undercontrolled" in childhood had elevated rates of alcohol dependence and alcohol problems in young adulthood. A group classified as "Inhibited" also had elevated scores for alcohol problems; this was true for boys but not for girls.

Studies with multiethnic samples of adolescents from the New York metropolitan area by Wills and colleagues (1996) have used closely spaced assessments to test a theoretical model of early onset and escalation based on temperament and self-control (e.g., planning ahead, waiting for rewards). Studies of escalation have shown that around 12 years of age, future escalators had a much higher overall risk loading compared with experimenters or abstainers, being elevated on variables such as life stress, maladaptive coping, and peer substance use, and lower on variables such as parental support and academic competence. Structural modeling analyses for early onset show temperament characteristics of activity level and negative emotionality are related to poor self-control, while (with relative independence) positive mood and attentional focusing are related to good self-control (e.g., Wills et al., 2001). Poor self-control influences substance use involvement and escalation of use through exposing adolescents to more life stress and deviant peer affiliations, whereas good self-control has protective effects through promoting better academic competence (e.g., Wills et al., 2001; Wills and Stoolmiller, 2002; Novak and Clayton, 2001). In later adolescence, self-control and coping motives for use moderate the transition from substance use to substance abuse; for example, impulsive persons show more substance-related problems at a given level of substance use (Wills et al., 2002). Similar findings with outcomes including early substance use and sexual behavior have been obtained in studies with samples of minority adolescents in the Southern US (e.g., Brody and Ge, 2001; Wills et al., 2003).

Pandina and Johnson (1999) and colleagues have used an elaborated stress-coping model with a large regional sample of adolescents, initially assessed when participants were 12, 15, or 18 years of age, and followed with 3-year intervals into young or middle adulthood. Personality variables of disinhibition and hostility in adolescence predicted alcohol problems in young adulthood (Curran et al., 1997). Adolescent indices of chronic stress, negative coping styles (e.g., dealing with problems through anger), and perceiving alcohol use as a coping mechanism predicted alcohol dependence in young adulthood (Johnson and Pandina, 2000). Persons with persistent problem drinking were initially elevated on disinhibition and other problem behaviors (e.g., destroying property), and this group showed much poorer functioning in adulthood (Bennett et al., 1999).

3.2. Social Learning Models

The Oregon Youth Study, initiated by Gerald Patterson and colleagues, used a sample of boys from high-risk neighborhoods, initially assessed in 4th grade and followed over time with periodic assessments. Results showed that association with deviant peers often occurred by 12 years of age and was predictable from early measures of poor parental discipline and monitoring practices, poor academic performance, and poor social skills in childhood (Dishion et al., 1991). Deviant peer associations in early adolescence were found to mediate the relation between family and peer factors in childhood and substance use at 18 years of age (Dishion et al., 1995), and peer associations accounted for growth over time in substance use, sexual risk taking, and criminal behavior (Patterson et al., 2000). Another study in Oregon, with youth initially assessed at 11–15 years of age, also found peer substance use and variables such as family conflict contributed to escalation of problem behavior, and peers' use in late adolescence was a predictor of participants' use in young adulthood (e.g., Andrews et al., 2002). Adolescent's early experimentation (particularly with cigarette smoking) influenced subsequent growth in substance use involvement (Duncan et al., 1998) and chronicity of alcohol use in adolescence was a predictor of a range of problems in young adulthood (Duncan et al., 1997).

Ellickson and colleagues have analyzed data from a large prevention study initiated with 7th graders in schools in California and Oregon; the participants were followed through high school and at age 23 years. Tucker, Ellickson, and Klein (2002) studied predictors of transitions to regular smoking in 12th grade; early substance experimentation and low grades were risk factors, while protective factors included parental support and living in a two-parent nuclear family. Growth mixture modeling (Tucker et al., 2003) found four trajectories of binge drinking over the period from early adolescence to young adulthood; drinking increasers were characterized from early ages as having more deviant behaviors (e.g., skipped school, stole from a store) and lower resistance efficacy for drug offers.

A study in Seattle by Hawkins and colleagues used a social development model (Catalano and Hawkins, 1996) and was based on a sample of participants initially assessed in 5th grade and followed with periodic assessments into young adulthood. Early onset of alcohol use was related to alcohol problems in late adolescence (Hawkins et al., 1997) and transition analyses indicated that eventual problem drinkers began to diverge from other individuals in alcohol use between elementary school and middle school (Guo et al., 2000). Risk factors for alcohol abuse/dependence in young adulthood included parental alcohol abuse, youth's externalizing and internalizing problems, living in a neighborhood with more trouble-making youth, more bonding to antisocial friends, more perceived rewards from alcohol, and relatively high levels of use in middle and high school (Guo et al., 2001). Protective factors included clear family rules, strong bonding to school, social skills for refusing alcohol offers, and moral beliefs.

3.3. High-Risk Samples

Several studies have tested theoretical models with children of substance-abusing parents, in view of the elevated risk attributable to family history (e.g., Windle, 1990). Chassin and colleagues (1993) have used a stress-coping model.

This research was based on two groups of adolescents who were 10.5–15.5 years of age at baseline; one group had a biological parent who was alcoholic, the other group was demographically-matched controls with no parental alcoholism. Structural modeling analyses of early use showed vulnerability pathways, with parental alcoholism related to more life stress and negative emotionality among children, which in turn were related to more affiliation with drug-using peers; there was a protective pathway through parents' monitoring of children's behavior. For alcohol abuse/dependence in young adulthood there were pathways from parental alcoholism to externalizing (but not internalizing) symptomatology and alcohol use in adolescence; parental antisocial personality had a direct effect to drug abuse/dependence (Chassin et al., 1999; Chassin et al., 2002). A study of similar design that began when children were 3–5 years of age was based on a multifactorial model of pathways to substance abuse (Zucker, 1994). This research finds the high-risk group scoring lower at young ages on cognitive indices such as abstract planning and attentional focusing (Puttler et al., 1998) and scoring higher on measures of undercontrol and behavior problems (Loukas et al., 2003).

Tarter and colleagues have utilized temperament and self-control constructs (Tarter et al., 1999) in a study being conducted in Pittsburgh with a group of children from families having a parent with a substance abuse disorder, and demographically-matched controls with no parental substance abuse. Participants were initially assessed at 10–12 years of age (Wave 1) and were followed at 2-year intervals. A series of reports from this project has related temperament and executive cognitive functioning (ECF) to intermediate variables such as peer interaction and negative affectivity (e.g., Shoal and Giancola, 2003). Giancola and Parker (2001) found that baseline scores for ECF and difficult temperament independently (in opposite directions) predicted aggression and deviant peer affiliations at Wave 2, which in turn both predicted drug use at Wave 3 (ages 14–16 years). Tarter et al. (2003) reported data from Wave 4 (17–19 years of age), utilizing a composite dysregulation score derived from earlier assessments based on difficult temperament, ECF, externalizing symptomatology, and disruptive classroom behavior. Dysregulation from Wave 1 predicted substance use disorder at Wave 3, and Wave 3 dysregulation discriminated substance abusers from nonabusers at Wave 4.

3.4. Minority Samples

The research previously discussed was typically based on predominantly Caucasian populations. In recent years, investigators have conducted longitudinal studies with samples of ethnic minorities. These have extended the generality of previous findings and have identified new variables, such as ethnic identity and racial discrimination, that have a significant role in substance use or nonuse (e.g., Gibbons et al., 2004).

Friedman and Glassman (2000) studied a sample drawn from the rolls of the National Collaborative Perinatal Project. The analytic sample was persons who were African-American and had data at ages 16 years, 24 years, and 26 years. For predicting duration/intensity of substance use at age 26, adolescent risk factors were mostly indices of the amount of time the participant or his/her friends spent in deviant or illegal activity. Protective factors were peers' involvement in conventional pursuits (e.g., Boy/Girl Scouts, studying to get good grades) and amount of leisure time spent alone rather than with friends. Family risk factors included parents having drug problems and being angry, unreliable or unavailable; a protective factor was that mother had helped the participant with school work during adolescence.

Zimmerman and Schmeelk-Cone (2003) studied a sample of African-American adolescents from urban schools. The participants were initially assessed in 9th grade (mean age 14.6 years) and were followed at yearly intervals, with a fifth wave conducted two years after high school. Baseline data showed school motivation was lower among those who were already using alcohol and marijuana. Results from multiwave analyses showed that low school motivation contributed to continued drug use. The reciprocal path was not found, but heavy alcohol and marijuana use in adolescence reduced the likelihood of school graduation.

Bryant et al. (2003) examined academic variables with a multiethnic national sample of public school students assessed at ages 14 years and 20 years. Predisposing factors for increase in substance (tobacco, alcohol, or marijuana) use included negative attitudes toward school, placing little value on education, having friends with corresponding attitudes, and having less support from parents for academics. Tests showed that effects of some risk factors on substance use (e.g., school misbehavior) were stronger among Caucasians, but in general the effects of academic involvement were similar for majority and minority students.

Research being conducted in rural North Carolina has participants who are predominantly Caucasian but the study includes a sizable group of American Indian participants. A sample screened for elevated risk was initially assessed at 9, 11, or 13 years of age and is being followed over time with yearly assessments. A report based on three waves of data showed cross-sectional associations of behavioral undercontrol disorders with substance use for both ethnic groups and both genders; associations for emotional disorders (anxiety and depression) were significant only among Caucasian girls. Having a disorder increased the likelihood of substance use, but some tests showed initial substance use (particularly tobacco) related to subsequent disorder; both types of effects were prominent among American Indians though some effects were also found among Caucasians (Federman et al., 1997). Boys with abuse/dependence at age 16 showed earlier onset of substance use whereas girls with abuse/dependence showed later onset, implying that they progressed to abuse more rapidly (Costello et al., 1999).

4. SUMMARY AND DISCUSSION

This chapter has discussed longitudinal studies conducted with a variety of populations and utilizing different approaches to recruitment of subjects and assessment of predictors. Each study had some limitations (though different ones across studies) along with strengths accruing from the population studied and the methods utilized. A number of findings are consistent across studies, despite variations in populations and methods. Thus longitudinal research provides a rich resource, providing knowledge that can be used to help shape the content of prevention programs aimed at deterring the onset or persistence of substance use problems.

A summary of predictors is presented in Table 1. The results were observed over intervals from 4–5 years to 25–30 years and were obtained across different indices of substance use. We emphasize that extensive involvement in substance use in adolescence is a risk factor for drug abuse and adverse consequences in work, health, and social domains at later ages.

4.1. Risk Factors

Family risk factors are familial history of substance abuse (or current parental or other adult abuse), parental psychological problems and antisociality, and low

Table 1. Summary of Risk and Protective Factors for Drug Abuse

Risk factors	Protective factors
• Parental substance use, abuse	• Emotional, instrumental family support, family rules and organization
• Parental anger, mental health problems, antisocial personality	• discipline and monitoring
• Low family attachment, family conflict	• Temperament: attentional focusing, positive emotionality
• Early onset of use	• Good self-control (e.g., planfulness, executive functioning)
• Temperament: activity level, negative emotionality	• Conventional attitudes (e.g., value on achievement)
• Poor self-control (e.g., impulsiveness, disinhibition)	• Perceived harmfulness of drugs
• Risk taking, sensation seeking	• Moral beliefs
• Deviance-prone, unconventional attitudes (e.g., tolerance for deviance)	• Resistance efficacy
• Life stress, racial discrimination	• Academic involvement
• Externalizing symptomatology	• Perceived control, self-esteem, ethnic identity
• Deviant peer affiliations	
• Motives for use	
• Availability of drugs	
• Neighborhood disorganization	
• Genetic factors	

attachment plus frequent conflict with parents. Individual factors include poor self-control, a tendency to seek out risks, and deviance-prone attitudes (e.g., rebelliousness, tolerance for deviance). Temperament dimensions such as activity and negative emotionality are risk factors for early onset, and early onset and high-intensity use during adolescence predict substance use problems in adulthood. Other factors are life stress, affiliating with deviant peers, having coping motives for drug use, and externalizing-type symptomatology. Environmental factors include neighborhood disorganization and availability of drugs. Genetic factors have been suggested recently but are not well understood (McGue, 1999; Tarter et al., 1999).

4.2. Protective Factors

Protective family factors are supportive relationships with parents together with consistent discipline and monitoring by them. Protective temperament characteristics (attentional focusing, positive emotionality) and good self-control reduce onset and reduce the impact of risk factors. Academic orientation is protective, including positive attitudes toward school, valuing achievement as a goal, and getting good grades. Having moral beliefs and viewing religion as important are inversely related to drug abuse, as are social skills that enable persons to resist pressures for substance use and other risky behaviors.

4.3. Models of Predictive Effects

It is evident that drug abuse has many predictors. How, then, do these factors interrelate so as to place individuals on trajectories toward or away from drug abuse? This question has not really been addressed in most of the studies, because the analyses typically tested only whether variables at one point predicted drug abuse outcomes at a subsequent point. Few studies have tested the flow of processes over time, determining how variables operate so as to "push" individual trajectories toward or away from adverse outcomes (Tarter and Vanyukov, 1994; Zucker, 1994). For example, it is likely that parental substance abuse has effects on family relationships and on children's affect and coping, which in turn have implications for their performance in school and the kinds of peers they hang out with. It is these intermediate processes that can lead to escalated use, but at present there is still relatively little understanding of mediation processes in liability for drug abuse (Wills and Yaeger, 2003). Several models have outlined how to conceptualize the flow of influences from earlier to later factors (Catalano and Hawkins, 1996; Rothbart and Ahadi, 1994; Tarter and Vanyukov, 1994; Wills and Dishion, 2004; Zucker, 1994), and these may be useful to persons who are designing further research or analyzing longitudinal data.

4.4.   Where Can Research Go from Here?

A number of variables have been identified that predict substance abuse over considerable time periods. Yet some issues are not well resolved in current studies and we think will likely be the focus in further research. One issue is that although a number of predictors have been identified, it is not always clear how the flow of effects from one level to another occurs (e.g., family history to family interaction, self-control to peer affiliations) and how downstream effects from one time to another operate (e.g., early adolescence to middle adolescence). Research is needed to help clarify how effects of distal factors are translated into impact on proximal factors so as to influence specific manifestations of substance use or abuse. Analyses testing both direct effects and indirect effects (Figure 1) would help to clarify the nature of predictive processes. Another aspect is that the unfolding of temporal relations between predictors and outcomes over time is sometimes unclear, so research using techniques such as growth modeling and trajectory analysis would be useful to clarify how variables affect each other over time (e.g., Chassin et al., 2002; White et al., 2001; Wills and Stoolmiller, 2002). Person-centered analytic approaches may help to integrate data on predictive effects, as it is likely that persons with persistent problem use differ systematically from both abstainers and moderate users on a number of variables (Schulenberg et al., 1996; Wills et al., 1996).

We think that research will increasingly be influenced by behavior genetic approaches, given the sizable genetic contributions noted for many aspects of substance use and abuse (e.g., Iacono et al., 1999; Rutter, 2002). It is likely that longitudinal studies will be advised to obtain genetic samples, and research will include analytic approaches to help understand how variation at the level of genes is translated into effects on patterns of behavior (i.e., mediation, McGue, 1999), and how expression of genetic effects is shaped by the environment in which development occurs (i.e., moderation, Dick et al., 2001). Where feasible, incorporation of physiological assessments such as stress reactivity, and physiological measures such as cortisol and other stress-related hormones, may help to provide a broadened perspective on risk and protective processes. This aspect of longitudinal research can be guided by theoretical models that help to understand how multiple levels of variables influence each other over time (Wills and Dishion, 2004).

Disclaimer. This work was supported by a Research Scientist Development Award K02 DA00252 from the National Institute on Drug Abuse (TAW), a Minority Supplement Award DA12623-S1, from the National Institute on Drug Abuse (CW), and grant R01 DA12623 from the National Institute on Drug Abuse (JAR).

REFERENCES

Andrews, J. A., Tildesley, E., Hops, H., and Li, F. (2002). The influence of peers on young adult substance use. *Health Psychology* 21, pp. 349–357.

Bachman, J. G., O'Malley, P. M., Schulenberg, J. E., Johnston, L. D., Bryant, A. L. and Merline, A. C. (2002). *The Decline of Substance Use in Young Adulthood.* Lawrence Erlbaum Associates, Mahwah, NJ.

Bennett, M. E., McCrady, B. S., Johnson, V., and Pandina, R. J. (1999). Problem drinking from young adulthood to adulthood. *Journal of Studies on Alcohol* 60, pp. 605–614.

Brody, G. H., and Ge, X. (2001). Linking parenting processes and self-regulation to alcohol use during early adolescence. *Journal of Family Psychology* 15(1), pp. 82–94.

Brook, D. W., Brook, J. S., Zhang, C., Cohen, P., and Whiteman, M. (2002). Drug use and the risk of major depressive disorder, alcohol dependence, and substance use disorders. *Archives of General Psychiatry* 59, pp. 1039–1044.

Brook, J., Richter, L., Whiteman, M., and Cohen, P. (1999). Consequences of adolescent marijuana use. *Genetic, Social, and General Psychology Monographs* 125, pp. 193–207.

Brook, J. S., Whiteman, M., Cohen, P., Shapiro, J., and Balka, E. (1995). Predicting late adolescent and young adult drug use: Childhood and adolescent precursors. *Journal of the American Academy of Child and Adolescent Psychiatry* 34, pp. 1230–1238.

Bryant, A. L., Schulenberg, J., O'Malley, P. M., Bachman, J. G., and Johnston, L. D. (2003). How academic achievement/attitudes relate to the course of substance use during adolescence: A longitudinal study. *Journal of Research on Adolescence* 13, pp. 361–397.

Caspi, A., Moffitt, T., Newman, D., and Silva, P. (1996). Behavioral observations at age 3 years predict adult psychiatric disorders. *Archives of General Psychiatry* 53, pp. 1033–1039.

Catalano, R. F., and Hawkins, J. D. (1996). The social development model: A theory of antisocial behavior. In J. D. Hawkins (Ed.), *Delinquency and Crime: Current Theories.* Cambridge University Press. New York, pp. 149–197.

Chassin, L. A., Pillow, D. R., Curran, P. J., Molina, B., and Barrera, M. (1993). Relation of parental alcoholism to early adolescent substance use: A test of three mediating mechanisms. *Journal of Abnormal Psychology* 102, pp. 3–19.

Chassin, L., Pitts, S. C., DeLucia, C., and Todd, M. (1999). A longitudinal study of children of alcoholics: Predicting young adult substance use disorders, anxiety, and depression. *Journal of Abnormal Psychology* 108, pp. 106–119.

Chassin, L., Pitts, S. C., and Prost, J. (2002). Binge drinking trajectories from adolescence to adulthood in a high-risk sample: Predictors and substance use outcomes. *Journal of Consulting and Clinical Psychology* 70, pp. 67–78.

Chen, K., and Kandel, D. (1995). Natural history of drug use from adolescence to the mid-thirties in a general population sample. *American Journal of Public Health, 85,* 41–47.

Cloninger, C. R. (1987). Neurogenetic adaptive mechanisms in alcoholism. *Science* 236, pp. 410–416.

Costello, E. J., Erkanli, A., Federman, E., and Angold, A. (1999). Development of psychiatric co-morbidity with substance abuse in adolescents: Effects of timing and sex. *Journal of Clinical Child Psychology* 28, pp. 298–311.

Curran, G., White, H. W., and Hansell, S. (1997). Predicting problem drinking: A test of a social learning model. *Alcoholism: Clinical and Experimental Research* 21, pp. 1379–1390.

Dick, D. M., Rose, R. J., Viken, R. J., Kaprio, J., and Koskenvuo, M. (2001). Exploring gene-environment interactions. *Journal of Abnormal Psychology* 110, pp. 625–632.

Dishion, T. J., Capaldi, D., Spracklen, K. M., and Li, F. (1995). Peer ecology of male adolescent drug use. *Development and Psychopathology* 7, pp. 803–824.

Dishion, T. J., Patterson, G. R., Stoolmiller, M., and Skinner, M. L. (1991). Family, school, and behavioral antecedents to early adolescent involvement with antisocial peers. *Developmental Psychology* 27, pp. 172–180.

Donovan, J. E., and Jessor, R. (1985). Structure of problem behavior in adolescence and young adulthood. *Journal of Consulting and Clinical Psychology* 53, pp. 890–904.

Donovan, J. E., Jessor, R., and Costa, F. M. (1991). *Beyond Adolescence: Problem Behavior and Young Adult Development.* Cambridge University Press, New York.

Duncan, S. C., Alpert, A., Duncan, T. E., and Hops, H. (1997). Adolescent alcohol use development and young adult outcomes. *Drug and Alcohol Dependence* 49, pp. 39–48.

Duncan, S., Duncan, T. E., and Hops, H. (1998). Progressions of cigarette, alcohol, and marijuana use in adolescence. *Journal of Behavioral Medicine* 21, pp. 375–388.

Ensminger, M. E., Juon, H. S., and Fothergill, K. E. (2002). Childhood and adolescent antecedents of substance use in adulthood. *Addiction* 97, pp. 833–844.

Federman, E. B., Costello, E. J., Angold, A., Farmer, E. M. Z., and Erkanli, A. (1997). Development of substance use and psychiatric comorbidity in White and American Indian young adolescents. *Drug and Alcohol Dependence* 44, pp. 69–78.

Friedman, A. S., and Glassman, K. (2000). Family and peer risk factors for drug abuse: A longitudinal study of an African American community sample. *Journal of Substance Abuse Treatment* 18, pp. 267–275.

Giancola, P. R., and Parker, A. M. (2001). A 6-year prospective study of pathways towards drug use in adolescent boys with and without a family history of a substance use disorder. *Journal of Studies on Alcohol* 62, pp. 166–178.

Gibbons, F. X., Gerrard, M., Cleveland, M. J., Wills, T. A., and Brody, G. H. (2004). Perceived discrimination and substance use in African-American parents and their children: A panel study. *Journal of Personality and Social Psychology* 86, pp. 517–529.

Guo, J., Collins, L. M., Hill, K. G., and Hawkins, J. D. (2000). Developmental pathways to alcohol abuse in young adulthood. *Journal of Studies on Alcohol* 61, pp. 799–808.

Guo, J., Hawkins, J. D., Hill, K. G., and Abbott, R. D. (2001). Childhood and adolescent predictors of alcohol abuse and dependence in young adulthood. *Journal of Studies on Alcohol* 62, pp. 754–762.

Harrison, P. A., Fulkerson, J. A., and Beebe, T. J. (1998). DSM-IV substance use disorder criteria for adolescents. *American Journal of Psychiatry* 155, pp. 486–492.

Hawkins, J. D., Graham, J. W., Maguin, E., Abbott, R., Hill, K. G., and Catalano, R. F. (1997). Exploring the effects of age of alcohol use initiation and psychosocial risk factors on subsequent alcohol misuse. *Journal of Studies on Alcohol* 58, pp. 280–290.

Iacono, W. G., Carlson, S. R., Taylor, J., Elkins, I. J., and McGue, M. (1999). Behavioral disinhibition and the development of substance use disorders: Findings from the Minnesota Twin Family Study. *Development and Psychopathology* 11, pp. 869–900.

Jessor, R., and Jessor, S. L. (1977). *Problem Behavior and Psychosocial Development.* Academic Press, New York.

Jessor, R., Turbin, M. S., and Costa, F. M. (1998). Protective factors in adolescent health behavior. *Journal of Personality and Social Psychology* 75, pp. 788–800.

Johnson, V., and Pandina, R. J. (2000). Alcohol problems among a community sample: Influences of stress, coping, and gender. *Substance Use and Misuse* 35, pp. 669–686.

Johnston, L. D., O'Malley, P. M., and Bachman, J. G. (2000). *National Survey Results on Drug Use from The Monitoring The Future Study, 1975–1999. Volume 1: Secondary School Students.* National Institute on Drug Abuse, Rockville, MD.

Kandel, D. B., Davies, M., Karus, D., and Yamaguchi, K. (1986). The consequences in young adulthood of adolescent drug use. *Archives of General Psychiatry* 43, pp. 746–754.

Kandel, D., Kessler, R. C., and Margulies, R. Z. (1978). Antecedents of adolescent initiation into stages of drug use. In D. B. Kandel (Ed.), *Longitudinal Research on Drug Use.* Wiley, New York, pp. 73–100.

Kandel, D., Yamaguchi, K., and Chen, K. (1992). Stages of progression in drug use from adolescence to adulthood. *Journal of Studies on Alcohol* 53, pp. 447–457.

Kellam, S. G., Brown, C. H., and Fleming, J. P. (1982). Social adaptation to first grade and teenage drug, alcohol and cigarette use. *Journal of School Health* 52, pp. 301–306.

Loukas, A., Zucker, R. A., Fitzgerald, H. E., and Krull, J. L. (2003). Trajectories of behavior problems among sons of alcoholics: Effects of parent psychopathology, family conflict, and child undercontrol. *Journal of Abnormal Psychology* 112, pp. 119–131.

Mâsse, L. C., and Tremblay, R. E. (1997). Behavior of boys in kindergarten and the onset of substance use during adolescence. *Archives of General Psychiatry* 54, pp. 62–68.

McGue, M. (1999). The behavioral genetics of alcoholism. *Current Directions in Psychological Science* 8, pp. 109–115.

Newcomb, M., and Bentler, P.M. (1988a). *Consequences of Adolescent Drug Use.* Sage Publications, Newbury Park, CA.

Newcomb, M. D., and Bentler, P. M. (1988b). Impact of adolescent drug use and social support on problems of young adults. *Journal of Abnormal Psychology* 97, pp. 64–75.

Newcomb, M. D., Chou, C-P., Bentler, P. M., and Huba, G. J. (1988). Motivations as predictors of changes in drug use. *Journal of Counseling Psychology* 35, pp. 426–438.

Newcomb, M. D., and Felix-Ortiz, M. (1992). Multiple protective and risk factors for drug use and abuse: Crosssectional and prospective findings. *Journal of Personality and Social Psychology* 63, pp. 280–296.

Newcomb, M. D., and Harlow, L. L. (1986). Life events and substance use among adolescents: Mediating effects of perceived loss of control and meaninglessness in life. *Journal of Personality and Social Psychology* 51, pp. 564–577.

Newcomb, M. D., Maddahian, E., and Bentler, P. M. (1986). Risk factors for drug use among adolescents: Concurrent and longitudinal analyses. *American Journal of Public Health* 76, pp. 525–531.

Novak, S. P., and Clayton, R. R. (2001). The influence of school environment and self-regulation on stages of cigarette smoking. *Health Psychology* 20, pp. 196–207.

Pandina, R. J., and Johnson, V. L. (1999). Why people use and abuse drugs: Progress toward a heuristic model. In: M. D. Glantz and C. R. Hartel (Eds.), *Drug abuse: Origins and Interventions.* American Psychological Association, Washington, D.C. pp. 119–147.

Patterson, G. R., Dishion, T. J., and Yoerger, K. (2000). Adolescent growth in new forms of problem behavior: Macro- and micro-peer dynamics. *Prevention Science* 1, pp. 3–13.

Pulkkinen, L., and Pitkänen, T. (1994). A prospective study of the precursors to problem drinking in young adulthood. *Journal of Studies on Alcohol* 55, pp. 578–587.

Puttler, L. I., Zucker, R. A., Fitzgerald, H. E., and Bingham, C. R. (1998). Behavioral outcomes among children of alcoholics during the early and middle childhood years. *Alcoholism: Clinical and Experimental Research* 22, pp. 1962–1972.

Rothbart, M. K., and Ahadi, S. A. (1994). Temperament and the development of personality. *Journal of Abnormal Psychology* 103, pp. 55–66.

Rutter, M. (2002). The interplay of nature, nurture, and developmental influences: The challenge ahead for mental health. *Archives of General Psychiatry* 59, pp. 996–1000.

Schulenberg, J., Wadsworth, K. N., O'Malley, P. M., Bachman, J. G., and Johnston, L. D. (1996). Risk factors for binge drinking during the transition to young adulthood: Pattern-centered approaches to change. *Developmental Psychology* 32, pp. 659–674.

Shoal, G. D., and Giancola, P. R. (2003). Negative affectivity and drug use in adolescent boys. *Journal of Personality and Social Psychology* 84, pp. 221–233.

Tarter, R. E., and Vanyukov, M. (1994). Alcoholism: A developmental disorder. *Journal of Consulting and Clinical Psychology* 62, pp. 1096–1107.

Tarter, R., Kirisci, L., Mezzich, A., Cornelius, J., Pajer, K., Vanyukov, M., Gardner, W., Blackson, T., and Clark, D. (2003). Neurobevioral disinhibition in childhood predicts early onset of substance use disorder. *American Journal of Psychiatry* 160, pp. 1078–1085.

Tarter, R., Vanyukov, M., Giancola, P., Dawes, M., Blackson, T., Mezzich, A., and Clark, D. (1999). Etiology of early age onset substance use disorder: A maturational perspective. *Development and Psychopathology* 11, pp. 657–683.

Tucker, J. S., Ellickson, P. L., and Klein, D. J. (2002). Five-year prospective study of risk factors for daily smoking among early nonsmokers and experimenters. *Journal of Applied Social Psychology* 32, pp. 1588–1603.

Tucker, J. S., Orlando, M., and Ellickson, P. L. (2003). Patterns of binge drinking trajectories from early adolescence to young adulthood. *Health Psychology 22,* pp. 79–87.

White, H. R., Xie, M., Thompson, W., Loeber, R., and Stouthamer-Loeber, M. (2001). Psychopathology as a predictor of adolescent drug use trajectories. *Psychology of Addictive Behaviors* 15, pp. 210–218.

Wills, T. A., Cleary, S. D., Filer, M., Shinar, O., Mariani, J., and Spera, K. (2001). Temperament, self-control, and early substance use. *Prevention Science* 2, pp. 145–163.

Wills, T. A., and Dishion, T. J. (2004). Temperament and adolescent substance use: A transactional analysis. *Journal of Clinical Child and Adolescent Psychology* 33, pp. 69–81.

Wills, T. A., Gibbons, F. X., Gerrard, M., Murry, V., and Brody, G. (2003). Family communication and religiosity related to substance use and sexual behavior in early adolescence. *Psychology of Addictive Behaviors* 17, pp. 312–323.

Wills, T. A., McNamara, G., Vaccaro, D., and Hirky, A. E. (1996). Escalated substance use: A longitudinal grouping analysis. *Journal of Abnormal Psychology* 105, pp. 166–180.

Wills, T. A., Sandy, J. M., and Yaeger, A. (2002). Moderators of the relation between substance use level and problems. *Journal of Abnormal Psychology* 111, pp. 3–21.

Wills, T. A., and Stoolmiller, M. (2002). The role of self-control in early escalation of substance use. *Journal of Consulting and Clinical Psychology* 70, pp. 986–997.

Wills, T. A., and Yaeger, A. M. (2003). Family factors and adolescent substance use: Models and mechanisms. *Current Directions in Psychological Science* 12, pp. 222–226.

Windle, M. (1990). Temperament and personality attributes of children of alcoholics. In M. Windle and J. S. Searles (Eds.), *Children of Alcoholics* (pp. 129–167). Guilford, New York.

Zimmerman, M. A., and Schmeelk-Cone, K. H. (2003). A longitudinal analysis of adolescent substance use and school motivation among African-American youth. *Journal of Research on Adolescence* 13, pp. 185–210.

Zucker, R. A. (1994). Pathways to alcohol problems: A developmental account of the contextual contributions to risk. In: R. A. Zucker, G. M. Boyd, and J. Howard (Eds.), *The Development of Alcohol Problems* (pp. 255–289). National Institute on Alcohol Abuse and Alcoholism, Rockville, MD.

13

Drug Abuse and the Spread of Infection: HIV and AIDS as an Example

Don C. Des Jarlais, Holly Hagan, and Samuel R. Friedman

DON C. DES JARLAIS • Beth Israel Medical Center
HOLLY HAGAN AND SAMUEL R. FRIEDMAN • National Development and Research Institutes (NDRI)

1. INTRODUCTION

Drug abusers, particularly those that inject (IDU), are more susceptible to a variety of infections and health problems as a result of the effects of the drugs themselves or drug purity level, the contaminants in the mix of the drugs, microbes in the injecting equipment or drug solution, or drug-related lifestyles or behaviors (e.g., accidents, homicides, suicides, or sexually transmitted diseases). The most important infection associated with injecting and the drug using lifestyle of the past two decades has been human immunodeficiency virus (HIV), the virus that causes AIDS. The global spread of illicit drug injection has meant that many countries are now trying to cope with the simultaneous epidemics of illicit drug injection and HIV among injecting drug users. For this reason this chapter will focus on the discussion of HIV infection and AIDS as an example of the health consequences of drug using behaviors and their prevention.

2. HIV INFECTION AMONG INJECTING DRUG USERS

From the 1960s through the 1980s, the practice of injecting illicit drugs spread throughout the United States, Western Europe, and Australia. By the 1990s, it was estimated that there were 5 million injecting drug users (IDUs) in the world, mostly in industrialized countries (Mann et al., 1992). Since then, injecting drug use has spread and current estimates suggest that there are now 13 million IDUs with 10 million of these located in developing or transitional countries (Stimson et al., 2004). Along with this increased number of IDUs, HIV has also spread to over 100 countries (Des Jarlais et al., 1996), a substantial increase over the 59 countries reported in 1989 (Des Jarlais and Friedman, 1989). In many countries the most common risk factor for HIV infection is injecting drug use either directly through the sharing of drug equipment or indirectly through unprotected sexual contact (Des Jarlais et al., 1989; Wright et al., 1994). Given the multiple ways in which HIV may spread to local populations of IDUs, it would be unrealistic to expect that any local population of IDUs will remain free of HIV.

2.1. Rapid Transmission of HIV among IDUs

The micro-transfusions that can occur when two or more persons inject with the same needle and syringe are relatively efficient mechanisms for transmitting

HIV. The "sharing" of needles and syringes has lead to extremely rapid transmission of HIV among IDUs, with the HIV seroprevalence rate (the percentage of IDUs infected with HIV) increasing from less than 10 percent to 40 percent or greater within a period of one to two years (Des Jarlais et al., 1992). New York City experienced the first epidemic of HIV among IDUs beginning in the late 1970s (Des Jarlais et al., 1989) and reaching 50 percent prevalence (half of the IDUs infected with HIV) by the early 1980s. This was followed by rapid spread in a number of Western European countries, particularly in Italy and Spain (Stimson et al., 1998). Bangkok, Thailand was the first city in a developing country to experience rapid spread of HIV among IDUs, with prevalence rates increasing from 2 percent in late 1988 to over 40 percent by late 1989 (Vanichseni et al., 2002). The most recent rapid spread of HIV among IDUs has occurred in Eastern Europe, Russia and the Newly Independent States (the former Soviet Union), and in parts of Asia, including China and Vietnam (UNAIDS/WHO, 2003)

This extremely rapid transmission of HIV among IDUs is believed to be due to: (a) lack of awareness of HIV and AIDS as a local threat; (b) restrictions on the availability and use of new injection equipment; and (c) mechanisms for rapid, efficient mixing within the local IDU population. Without an awareness of AIDS as a local threat, IDUs are likely to use each other's equipment very frequently. Indeed, prior to an awareness of HIV and AIDS, the sharing of previously used equipment was seen as an act of solidarity among IDUs or as a service for which one may legitimately charge a small fee.

There are various types of legal restrictions that can reduce the availability of sterile injection equipment leading to increased multi-person use ("sharing") of drug injection equipment. In some jurisdictions, medical prescriptions are required for the purchase of needles and syringes. Possession of needles and syringes can also be criminalized as "drug paraphernalia," putting users at risk of arrest if needles and syringes are found in their possession. In some jurisdictions drug users have also been prosecuted for possession of drugs based on the minute quantities of drugs that remain in a needle and syringe after it has been used to inject drugs. In addition the possible legal restrictions on the availability of sterile injection equipment, the actual practices of pharmacists and police can create important limits. Even if laws permit sales of needles and syringes without prescriptions, pharmacists may choose not to sell without prescriptions, or not to sell to anyone who "looks like a drug user." Similarly, police may harass drug users found carrying injection equipment even if there are no laws criminalizing the possession of narcotics paraphernalia.

"Shooting galleries" (places where IDUs can rent injection equipment, which is then returned to the gallery owner for rental to other IDUs), "dealer's works" (injection equipment kept by a drug seller, which can be lent to successive drug purchasers), and "hit doctors" (persons, often drug users themselves, who inject others, typically using the same needle and syringe for successive clients) are all examples of situations that provide rapid, efficient mixing within an IDU population. The "mixing" is rapid in that many IDUs may use the gallery or the dealer's injection equipment within very short periods of time. Several studies have indicated that the infectiousness of HIV is many times greater in the 2–3 month period after initial infection compared to the long "latency" period between initial infection and the development of severe immunosuppression. (Jacquez et al., 1994). Thus, the concentration of new infections in these settings may synergistically interact with continued mixing and lead to highly infectious IDUs transmitting HIV to large numbers of other drug injectors. "Efficient" mixing refers to the sharing of drug injection equipment with little or no restriction upon who shares with whom. Thus, efficient mixing serves to spread HIV across potential social boundaries, such as friendship groups, which otherwise might have served to limit transmission.

3.   PREVENTING HIV AMONG IDUS

While there is a clear possibility of rapid transmission of HIV among IDUs, there is also a clear possibility of greatly reducing HIV transmission among IDUs. The common stereotype that IDUs are not at all concerned about health led to initial expectations that they would not change their behavior because of AIDS. In sharp contrast to these expectations, reductions in risk behavior and in HIV incidence (the rate of new HIV infections) were observed among IDU participants in a wide variety of early prevention programs, including outreach/bleach distribution (Thompson et al., 1990; Wiebel et al., 1990), "education only" (Jackson and Rotkiewicz, 1987; Ostrow, 1989), drug abuse treatment (Blix and Gronbladh, 1988), syringe exchange (Buning et al., 1988), increased over-the-counter sales of injection equipment (Espinoza et al., 1988; Goldberg et al., 1988), and HIV counseling and testing (Cartter et al., 1990; Higgins et al., 1991).

It is also important to note that there is evidence that IDUs will reduce HIV risk behavior even in the absence of any specific prevention program. IDUs in New York City reported risk reduction prior to the implementation of any formal HIV prevention programs. IDUs had learned about AIDS through the mass media and the oral-communication networks within the drug-injecting population (Friedman et al., 1987; Selwyn et al., 1987) and the illicit market in sterile injection equipment had expanded to provide additional equipment. (Des Jarlais et al., 1985).

3.1.   Effective Programs for Reducing HIV Risk Behavior among IDUs

While risk reduction among IDUs has occurred in response to a wide variety of specific programs, the currently available evidence provides strong support for the effectiveness of three types of programs: community outreach, syringe exchange, and methadone maintenance treatment (National Institutes of Health, 1997). Table 1 summarizes an evaluation study showing strong effects of each of these types of programs. In each of these examples, HIV incidence was used as

Table 1. Examples of Effective HIV Prevention Programs for Injecting Drug Users

Intervention	Reference	Sample	Intervention	Outcome
Community/ Street Outreach	(Wiebel, 1996)	641 HIV negative Chicago IDUs	Indigenous Leader Outreach model— ex-addicts providing HIV education and counseling	• Decline in injection risk behavior from 100% to 14% reporting equipment sharing • Decrease in HIV seroconversion rate: 8.4/100 PY (1988) vs. 2.4/100 PY (1992)
Sterile Syringe Access	(Des Jarlais et al., in press)	IDUs entering drug treatment	New York City syringe exchange programs	• HIV incidence declined from 3.55/100 PY to 0.77/100 PY
Drug Treatment Programs	(Metzger et al., 1993)	255 IDUs (152 in-treatment and 103 out-of-treatment)	Outpatient methadone treatment in Philadelphia	• Over 18 months, 3.5% of in-treatment IDUs seroconverted to HIV positive vs. 22% of out-of-treatment subjects

the outcome measure, the HIV incidence rate in the local community was generally high, and the comparison group was receiving relatively few HIV prevention services.

3.1.1. Community/Street Outreach Programs

These programs involve disseminating HIV/AIDS information within the local IDU population. Such programs typically use ex- or current drug users as "peer educators" who are first trained and then sent back into the community to educate others. These peer educators typically have good knowledge of the local IDU population and have existing trusting relationships with many IDUs. The peer educators are often hired as full time staff of the project. Two excellent examples of alternative uses of peer educators are described by Broadhead et al. (1998) and Latkin et al. (1998, 2003).

Community outreach/peer education programs appear to be an excellent method for disseminating information about HIV and AIDS to IDUs. These programs take advantage of naturally occurring communication channels and social networks among illicit drug users and provide opportunities for the development of new social norms regarding risk behaviors and for social reinforcement of risk reduction. A limitation of many community outreach/peer education programs is the failure to provide the supplies (sterile needles and syringes, condoms) needed for practicing safer behavior.

3.1.2.   Syringe Exchange Programs

The fundamental principle of syringe exchange programs is the exchanging of new (sterile) needles and syringes for used needles and syringes. This both provides for safe disposal of potentially HIV contaminated injection equipment and increases the ability of the clients to practice safer injection. Syringe exchange operations have evolved over the twenty years since the first program was begun in Amsterdam in 1984. The general direction has been towards more services and towards more "user friendly services" (Des Jarlais et al., 1995). Variations have developed on the original "one for one" exchanging of needles and syringes and many programs believe that no drug user who comes to the exchange should leave without a sufficient supply of clean needles and syringes. Thus, some programs will provide a "two for one" exchange for up to five syringes or simply give an extra number of clean needles and syringes in addition to the exchanged needles and syringes.

"Secondary exchanging" has also developed as an important method for getting more clean needles and syringes to more drug users. Some drug users will exchange not only for their own personal use but also for friends and acquaintances even up to hundreds of needles and syringes in a single visit. These secondary exchangers can be considered as unpaid extended staff of the program. Some programs have also adopted "independently scheduled exchange services" in which a drug user will contact program staff and arrange a meeting at a convenient discrete location in order to conduct exchange (Des Jarlais and Shimizu, 2003). Both the secondary exchanging and the independently scheduled exchanging permit expansion of exchange services beyond the set hours and locations of the primary program. These approaches can also be seen as integration of syringe exchange into the drug user community and as drug users taking on more responsibility for facilitating safer injection within the community.

Over time syringe programs have become important sites for providing a wide variety of non-exchange services to drug users through both on-site services and referrals to other services. The most commonly offered services are: information about safer sex and provision of condoms, voluntary HIV counseling and testing, and referrals to drug abuse treatment. In the United States, the provision of additional services is strongly related to the source of funding. To date, there has been no federal government funding for syringe exchange programs, despite numerous evaluations which concluded that syringe exchange programs are effective in reducing HIV transmission among IDUs and that syringe exchange programs do not lead to any increase in drug abuse (Normand et al., 1995)

While syringe exchange programs have almost always been effective in reducing HIV risk behavior, there have been a few programs that clearly did not control HIV transmission within the local population of IDUs. In Vancouver and Montreal, local IDUs were primarily injecting cocaine which, because of associated binge injecting, required more clean needles and syringes than were supplied. Recognition of this need by increasing the numbers of syringes exchanged had led to a reduction in HIV transmission in both cities (Strathdee et al., 1998).

3.1.3.   Long-Term Drug Abuse Treatment Programs

While peer education programs and syringe exchange programs reduce HIV risk behavior through providing for safer injection (injecting without sharing of needles and syringes). Drug abuse treatment programs work to reduce HIV risk through the reduction of drug injecting. Reducing drug use provides numerous other benefits besides reduction in HIV risk to both the individual drug user and to the community as a whole.

While there are a variety of types of drug abuse treatment—methadone maintenance, residential drug free and outpatient drug free and self-help recovery programs—that can reduce drug use in general and drug use in particular, the evidence for methadone maintenance is the strongest (Des Jarlais et al., 2004a, Avants et al., 2004; Metzger et al., 1993). Drug abuse treatment does hold considerable appeal as a means of reducing HIV risk, but there are also important limitations on its effectiveness. First, some types of "treatment," such as forced detoxification, do not show any long-term effectiveness, with relapse rates of approximately 90 percent or more. Second, not all drug users are psychologically ready to enter and benefit from drug abuse treatment. Third, drug abuse treatment is relatively expensive, and few countries, including developed countries, provide treatment on a scale large enough to impact HIV transmission in the community.

4.   INTEGRATING MULTIPLE HIV PREVENTION PROGRAMS FOR IDUS

Assisting drug injectors to practice safer injection and providing drug abuse treatment to reduce drug injection per se are complementary strategies. One of the most important lessons of the early outreach programs was that the process of teaching drug injectors how to practice safer injection uncovered a previously hidden demand for entry into drug abuse treatment. This unexpected demand for drug abuse treatment led to a program in which New Jersey outreach workers distributed vouchers that could be redeemed for no-cost detoxification treatment (Jackson and Rotkiewicz, 1987). Over 95 percent of the vouchers were redeemed by drug users entering treatment, many of whom had never before been in drug abuse treatment. There are also examples of syringe exchange programs that have become important sources of referral to drug abuse treatment programs. (For details see O'Keefe et al., 1991; Hagan et al., 1994; and, Des Jarlais and Shimizu, 2003). However, there is relatively little evidence of referrals being made from drug abuse treatment programs to syringe exchange programs although in some U.S. programs, clients are provided information about syringe exchange programs in the local area, and there are some European programs that offer both syringe exchange and drug abuse treatment at the same sites.

4.1. Limitations on HIV Risk Reduction

While there are many types of programs that reduce risk behavior among IDUs, there is no program or set of programs that have eliminated HIV risk behavior in any population. The term "residual risk behaviors" has been used to denote risk behavior remaining in a population after multiple prevention programs have been implemented on a large (public health level) scale (Des Jarlais and Friedman, 1998). In Amsterdam, for example, the percentage of IDUs reporting receptive sharing (injecting with a needle or syringe use by another person) had stabilized at approximately 30 percent (van Ameijden and Coutinho, 1998) while in other cities, receptive sharing has stabilized at between 14 percent and 20 percent. (Nelson et al., 2002; Braine et al., under review; Des Jarlais, 2002; Drummond et al., 2002; Des Jarlais et al., 2004).

4.1.1. Preventing Epidemics of HIV among Populations of IDUs

Current programs for reducing HIV transmission among IDUs should be considered highly effective at the individual level in that very large numbers of IDUs will adopt "safer" injection practices but not perfect as a substantial minority of IDUs will continue to engage in injection risk behavior after exposure to the programs. This leads to the question of the effectiveness of the programs at the community level. Can such programs prevent epidemics of HIV among IDUs or do the programs merely slow down and reduce the size of such epidemics? There is now over fifteen years of experience showing that these programs can prevent HIV epidemics among IDUs. There are a number of cities (Des Jarlais et al., 1995) and countries such as the United Kingdom (Stimson, 1995) and Australia (Wodak and Lurie, 1996) where HIV infection has been limited to less than 5 percent of the IDU population and the rates of new HIV infections are less than 1 percent per year. These examples share three common characteristics (Des Jarlais et al., 1995): prevention efforts were begun early, while HIV prevalence was 5 percent or less; trusted communication was established between health workers and the local community of IDUs (often through outreach efforts); and, IDUs had very good access to sterile injection equipment (through syringe exchange or pharmacy sales without much police interference of IDUs access to and use of the sterile injection equipment). In addition, HIV prevention programs need to adapt to changes in the local situation. This was the problem in Vancouver, where the local inject-ing practices switched from heroin to cocaine use. Persons injecting heroin will typically inject once every four hours at most while cocaine injectors frequently binge, injecting every 15 or 20 minutes until the supply of the drug is exhausted. If binge injecting occurs in a group setting, then either very large numbers of needles and syringes will be needed, or substantial amounts of sharing are likely to occur within the group. Initially, the numbers of syringes distributed by the local syringe exchange program in Vancouver were not sufficient to contain HIV transmission with the change to cocaine as the primary drug.

Thus, while it clearly is possible to prevent HIV epidemics among IDUs, the prevention programs need to be implemented on a sufficiently large scale and adapted to any changes in local drug use practices.

4.1.2. Bringing High HIV Prevalence Epidemics under Control

Once HIV seroprevalence reaches high levels (30 percent or more) in a population of IDUs, prevention of new HIV infections becomes much more challenging. With many IDUs capable of transmitting the virus, continued high rates of risk behavior can drive HIV seroprevalence to 80 percent to 90 percent or higher. (UNAIDS/WHO, 2003). This represents saturation levels of HIV in the local IDU population.

A brief survey of the current status of high servoprevalence epidemics among IDUs in developed countries shows both the self-perpetuating nature of these epidemics and some indications that, over long time periods, it may be possible to bring such epidemics under control. It is important to note that all of these areas have implemented multiple prevention programs, including legal access to sterile injection equipment, some form of community outreach and drug abuse treatment. For more information on the experiences of Canada see Hankins et al., 2002; Craib et al., 2003; and Spittal ct al., 2002; for Western Europe, European Centre for the Epidemiological Monitoring of AIDS, 2002; Perez et al., 2002; Broers, et al., 1998; and, Robertson, 1998; and, thc United States, Nelson et al., 2002; Quan et al., 2002; Braine et al., in preparation; Heimer and Singer, 2003.

New York City may provide the most dramatic example of the possibility of bringing a high seroprevalence epidemic under control. HIV was introduced into the IDU population in New York in the mid-1970s spreading rapidly during the late 1970s and early 1980s, reaching greater than 50 percent prevalence (Des Jarlais et al., 1989). Risk reduction/behavior change began shortly after AIDS was discovered in IDUs. News media coverage and social network communications lead to a widespread awareness of AIDS, how it was transmitted, and increased use of sterile injection equipment (Des Jarlais et al., 1985). Prevalence then stabilized at approximately 50 percent and incidence at approximately 5 percent per year (Des Jarlais et al., 1994). In the early 1990s, HIV prevention programs for IDUs were greatly expanded and the experience has become one of the most important success stories in HIV prevention for IDUs. Since the early 1990s, HIV incidence among

IDUs has declined from 5/100 person-years (py) to 1-2/100 py, and prevalence has declined from 50 percent to approximately 15 percent (Des Jarlais et al., 1994, 1998, 2004b).

The current evidence does suggest that it may be possible to bring large, high seroprevalence HIV epidemics under control. At best, however, this is a long-term process, with incidence falling below the rate at which HIV seropositives are lost to the active drug using population. Clearly, it is highly preferable to prevent the initial epidemics rather than trying to control them afterwards.

4.1.3. Preventing Sexual Transmission of HIV from IDUs to Non-Injecting Sexual Partners

While there is highly consistent evidence that IDUs will make large changes in their injection risk behavior in response to concerns about AIDS, changes in sexual behavior appear to be much more modest compared to injection risk behavior (Friedman et al., 1993). A recent meta-analysis of programs to reduce sexual risk behavior among drug users showed that these programs have an average "modest" effect that was statistically significant, but that the statistical significance of this effect came from the small number of studies that compared an intervention condition to no intervention condition (Des Jarlais and Semaan, 2002).

In general, IDUs appear more likely to make risk-reduction efforts (reduced numbers of partners, increased use of condoms) for "casual" sexual relationships rather than in "primary" sexual relationships (Friedman et al., 1993). The reasons for the difficulties in changing the sexual behavior of IDUs have not been fully clarified, but the problem appears in many different cultural settings, including IDUs in Asia, Europe, and South America, as well as in the United States (Ball et al., 1994). To place the problem in perspective, however, IDUs have undoubtedly changed their sexual risk behavior more than non-injecting heterosexuals in the United States as a whole (Laumann et al., 1994). One factor that appears to be important in reducing sexual risk behavior among IDUs is an altruistic desire to avoid transmitting HIV to a non-injecting sexual partner (Vanichseni et al., 1993; Friedman et al., 1994; European Centre for the Epidemiological Monitoring of AIDS, 2002). However, the type of drug used greatly influences behavior so that the use of crack cocaine is often associated with high frequencies of unsafe sexual behaviors and therefore has become an important risk factor for infection with HIV (Edlin et al., 1994).

It is also worth noting that additional strategies are needed for increasing safer sex among IDUs who engage in male-with-male sexual activities as they serve as a bridge between non drug-injecting men who engage in male-with-male sex and the larger IDU population. In many areas of the United States, HIV seroprevalence among men who engage in male-with-male sex is substantially higher than among exclusively heterosexual IDUs (Chiasson et al., 1991; Maslow et al., 2002). There are indications of a re-emergence of high-risk sexual behavior among men who have sex with men in the U.S. and Western Europe (Bluthenthal et al., 2001; Stolte et al., 2000). If high rates of unsafe sex should re-occur among men who have sex with men in the United States and other developed countries, this could lead to more HIV infection among IDU men who engage in male-with-male sex, followed by more transmission from these men to other IDUs.

Once HIV prevalence reaches a high level (30 percent or greater) in a local population of IDUs, transmission to non-injecting sexual partners is almost certain to become a substantial problem. The extent of that problem depends upon a variety of factors such as the numbers of IDUs who have regular sexual partners who do not inject drugs and the rate of partner change in these relationships, the frequency with which IDUs engage in commercial sex work, the frequency with which IDUs purchase commercial sex, and the extent of commercial sex work in the society as a whole. The extent of condom use and the presence of sexually transmitted diseases that facilitate HIV transmission (such as syphilis) can also greatly increase HIV transmission from IDUs to non-injecting sexual partners and then to additional persons who do not inject drugs (Saidel et al., in press).

Of great concern is whether HIV among IDUs may initiate a self-sustaining heterosexual transmission epidemic. This appears to have occurred in conjunction with the crack cocaine epidemic in several US cities (Edlin et al., 1994) and in the state of Manipur, India (Manipur State AIDS Control Society, 2002). The recent rapid spread of HIV among IDUs in Russia and Eastern Europe and in China (UNAIDS/WHO, 2003), has created the possibility that this will be followed by large, self-sustaining heterosexual transmission epidemics in those countries.

5.   CONCLUSION

HIV infection can be prevented without requiring the cessation of injecting drug use. This potential separation of a severe adverse potential consequence of drug use from the drug use itself has encouraged analysis of other areas in which adverse consequences of drug use might be reduced without requiring cessation of drug use. Examples would include vaccination of drug users for hepatitis A and B, and providing naloxone to drug users so that they can revive their peers from overdoses.

The ability of many IDUs to modify their behavior to reduce the chances of HIV infection has also led to new consideration of drug users as both concerned about their health and as capable of acting on that concern (without denying the compulsive nature of drug addiction). These ideas have formed much of the basis for what has been termed the "harm reduction" perspective on psychoactive drug use (Bluthenthal et al., 1998; Brettle, 1991; Des Jarlais et al., 1993; Des Jarlais, 1995; Heather et al., 1993; Sherman and Latkin, 2002). This perspective emphasizes the pragmatic need to reduce harmful consequences of psychoactive drug use while acknowledging that completely eliminating psychoactive drug use and abuse is not likely to be feasible in the foreseeable future. This perspective can be applied to both licit (alcohol, nicotine) as well as illicit psychoactive drugs and can readily be adapted to new developments. There are many pragmatic steps that can be taken to reduce social harms associated with licit drugs such as enforcement of laws to reduce drunken driving and raising taxes on nicotine products to reduce use by youth. Given current biochemistry technology and the globalization of trade in licit and illicit drugs, we must be prepared for the emergence of new drug related problems from new "designer" drugs to new infectious diseases among drug users.

REFERENCES

Avants, S. K., Margolin, A., Usubiaga, M. H., and Doebrick, C. (2004). Targeting HIV-related outcomes with intravenous drug users maintained on methadone: A randomized clinical trial of a harm reduction group therapy. *Journal of Substance Abuse Treatment 26*(2), pp. 67–78.

Ball, A., Des Jarlais, D. C., Donoghoe, M., Friedman, S. R., Goldberg, D., Hunter, G. M., Stimson, G. V., and Wodak, A. (1994). *Multi-Centre Study on Drug Injecting and Risk of HIV Infection*: Geneva: World Health Organization, Programme on Substance Abuse.

Blix, O. and Gronbladh, L. (1988). *AIDS and IV Heroin Addicts: The Preventive Effect of Methadone Maintenance in Sweden*. Paper presented at the Fourth International Conference on AIDS, Stockholm, Sweden.

Bluthenthal, R., Kral, A., Lorvick, J., Erringer, E., and Edlin, B. (1998). Harm reduction and needle exchange programs. *Lancet 351*(9118), pp. 1819–1820.

Bluthenthal, R., Kral, A., Gee, L., Lorvick, J., Moore, L., Srol, K., and Edlin, B. (2001). Trends in HIV seroprevalence and risk among gay or bisexual men who inject drugs in San Francisco, 1998 to 2000. *Journal of Acquired Immune Deficiency Syndrome 14*, pp. 264–269.

Braine, N., Des Jarlais, D. C., Zadoretzky, C., Goldblatt, C., and Turner, C. (Under review). HIV risk behavior among amphetamine injectors at US syringe exchange programs.

Brettle, R. P. (1991). HIV and harm reduction for injection drug users. *AIDS 5*, pp. 125–136.

Broadhead, R. S., Heckathorn, D. D., Weakliem, D. L., Anthony, D. L., Madray, H., Mills, R. J., and Hughes, J. J. (1998). Harnessing peer networks as an instrument for AIDS prevention: Results from a peer driven intervention. *Public Health Reports 113* Suppl 1, pp. 42–57.

Broers, B., Junet, C., Bourquin, M., Deglon, J. J., Perrin, L., & Hirschel, B. (1998). Prevalence and incidence of HIV, hepatitis B and C among drug users on methadone maintenance treatment in Geneva between 1988 and 1995. *AIDS 12*(15), pp. 2059–2066.

Buning, E. C., Hartgers, C., Verster, A. D., van Santen, G. W., and Coutinho, R. A. (1988). *The Evaluation of the Needle/Syringe Exchange in Amsterdam*. Paper presented at the IV International Conference on AIDS, Stockholm, Sweden.

Cartter, M. L., Petersen, L. R., Savage, R. B., and Donagher, J. (1990). Providing HIV counseling and testing services in methadone maintenance programs. *AIDS 4*(5), pp. 463–465.

Chiasson, M. A., Stoneburner, R. L., Hildebrandt, D. S., Ewing, W. E., Telzak, E. E., and Jaffe, H. W. (1991). Heterosexual transmission of HIV-1 associated with the use of smokable freebase cocaine (crack). *AIDS 5*, pp. 1121–1126.

Craib, K. J. P., Spittal, P. M., Wood, E., Laliberte, N., Hogg, R. S., Li, K., Heath, K., Tyndall, M. W., O'Shaughnessy, M. V., and Schechter, M. T. (2003). Risk factors for elevated HIV incidence among Aboriginal injection drug users in Vancouver. *Canadian Medical Association Journal* 168(1), pp. 19–24.

Des Jarlais, D. C. (1995). Harm reduction—a framework for incorporating science into drug policy. *American Journal of Public Health* 85(1), pp. 10–12.

Des Jarlais, D. C. (2002). *The state of syringe exchange in the known universe.* Paper presented at the 12th North American Syringe Exchange Convention, Albuquerque, NM.

Des Jarlais, D. C. and Friedman, S. R. (1989). AIDS and IV Drug Use. *Science* 245, pp. 578–579.

Des Jarlais, D. C. and Friedman, S. R. (1998). Fifteen years of research on preventing HIV infection among injecting drug users: What we have learned, what we have not learned, what we have done, what we have not done. *Public Health Reports* 113(Suppl 1), pp. 182–188.

Des Jarlais, D. C., and Semaan, S. (2002). HIV prevention research: Cumulative knowledge or accumulating studies? *Journal of Acquired Immune Deficiency Syndrome* 30(Suppl 1), pp. S1–S7.

Des Jarlais, D. C., and Shimizu, S. (2003). *2003 Evaluation Report: Hawaii Statewide Syringe Exchange Program.* Honolulu: Chow (Community Health Outreach Work) Project.

Des Jarlais, D. C., Friedman, S. R., and Hopkins, W. (1985). Risk reduction for the acquired immunodeficiency syndrome among intravenous drug users. *Annals of Internal Medicine* 103, pp. 755–759.

Des Jarlais, D. C., Friedman, S. R., Novick, D., Sotheran, J. L., Thomas, P., Yancovitz, S., Mildvan, D., Weber, J., Kreck, M. J., Maslansky, R., Bartelme, S., Spira, T., and Marmor, M. (1989). HIV-1 infection among intravenous drug users in Manhattan, New York City, from 1977 through 1987. *Journal of the American Medical Association* 261, pp. 1008–1012.

Des Jarlais, D. C., Friedman, S. R., Choopanya, K., Vanichseni, S., and Ward, T. P. (1992). International epidemiology of HIV and AIDS among injecting drug users. *AIDS* 6, pp. 1053–1068.

Des Jarlais, D. C., Friedman, S. R., and Ward, T. P. (1993). Harm reduction: A public health response to the AIDS epidemic among injecting drug users. *Annual Review of Public Health* 14, pp. 413–450.

Des Jarlais, D. C., Friedman, S. R., Sotheran, J. L., Wenston, J., Marmor, M., Yancovitz, S. R., Frank, B., Beatrice, S., and Mildvan, D. (1994). Continuity and change within an HIV epidemic: Injecting drug users in New York City, 1984 through 1992. *Journal of the American Medical Association* 271(2), pp. 121–127.

Des Jarlais, D., Hagan, H., Friedman, S., Friedman, P., Goldberg, D., Frischer, M., Green, S., Tunving, K., Ljungberg, B., Wodak, A., Ross, M., Purchase, D., Millson, M., and Myers, T. (1995). Maintaining low HIV seroprevalence in populations of injecting drug users. *Journal of the American Medical Association* 274(15), pp. 1226–1231.

Des Jarlais, D. C., Stimson, G. V., Hagan, H., Perlman, D., Choopanya, K., Bastos, F. I., and Friedman, S. R. (1996). Emerging infectious diseases and the injection of illicit psychoactive drugs. *Current Issues in Public Health* 2, pp. 102–137.

Des Jarlais, D. C., Perlis, T., Friedman, S. R., Deren, S., Chapman, T. F., Sotheran, J. L., Tortu, S., Beardsley, M., Paone, D., Torian, L. V., Beatrice, S. T., DeBernardo, E., Monterroso, E., and Marmor, M. (1998). Declining seroprevalence in a very large HIV epidemic: injecting drug users in New York City, 1991 to 1996. *American Journal of Public Health* 88(12), pp. 1801–1806.

Des Jarlais, D. C., Hagan, H., and Friedman, S. R. (2004a). Epidemiology and emerging public health perspectives. In: Lowinson, J., Millman, R. B. and Ruiz, P. (Eds.), *Substance Abuse: A Comprehensive Textbook 4e.* Lippincott Williams & Wilkins, New York.

Des Jarlais, D. C., Perlis, T., Arasteh, K., Hagan, H., Milliken, J., Braine, N., Yancovitz, S., Mildvan, D., Perlman, D., Maslow, C., and Friedman, S. R. (2004b). "Informed altruism" and "partner restriction" in the reduction of HIV infection in injecting drug users entering detoxification treatment in New York City, 1990–2001. *Journal of Acquired Immune Deficiency Syndrome* 35(2), pp. 158–166.

Des Jarlais, D. C., Perlis, T., Arasteh, K., Torian, L. V., Beatrice, S., Milliken, J., Mildvan, D., Yancovitz, S., and Friedman, S. R. (in press). STARHS testing for HIV incidence among injecting drug users in New York City, 1999–2002: Reduced incidence associated with expansion of syringe exchange programs. *American Journal of Public Health.*

Drummond, M., Health Outcomes International PTY LTD and the National Centre for HIV Epidemiology and Clinical Research (2002). *Return on Investment in Needle and Syringe Programs in Australia*: Commonwealth Department of Health and Aging.

Edlin, B. R., Irwin, K. L., and Faruque, S. (1994). Intersecting epidemics: Crack cocaine use and HIV infection among inner-city young adults. *New England Journal of Medicine* 331, pp. 1422–1427.

Espinoza, P., Bouchard, I., Ballian, P., and Polo DeVoto, J. (1988). *Has the Open Sale of Syringes Modified the Syringe Exchanging Habits of Drug Addicts?* Paper presented at the IV International Conference on AIDS, Stockholm, Sweden.

European Centre for the Epidemiological Monitoring of AIDS. (1996). *First Quarterly Report*. World Health Organization, Geneva.

European Centre for the Epidemiological Monitoring of AIDS. (2002). *Annual report on the state of the drugs problem in the European Union and Norway*. Luxembourg: European Monitoring Centre for Drugs and Drug Addiction.

Friedman, S. R., Des Jarlais, D. C., Sotheran, J. L., Garber, J., Cohen, H., and Smith, D. (1987). AIDS and self-organization among intravenous drug users. *International Journal of the Addictions* 22, pp. 201–219.

Friedman, S. R., Des Jarlais, D. C., and Ward, T. P. (1993). Overview of the History of the HIV Epidemic among Drug Injectors. In: B. S. Brown, B.S., Beschner, G.M., and National AIDS Research Consortium (Eds.), *Handbook on Risk of AIDS: Injection Drug Users and Sexual Partners*, Greenwood Press, Westport, CT, pp. 3–15.

Friedman, S. R., Jose, B., Neaigus, A., Goldstein, M., Curtis, R., Ildefonso, G., Mota, P., and Des jarlais, D.C. (1994). Consistent condom use in relationships between seropositive injecting drug users and sex partners who do not inject drugs. *AIDS* 8, pp. 357–361.

Goldberg, D., Watson, H., Stuart, F., Miller, M., Gruer, L., and Follett, E. (1988). *Pharmacy supply of needles and syringes-the effect on spread of HIV in intravenous drug misusers*. Paper presented at the Fourth International Conference on AIDS, Stockholm, Sweden.

Hagan, H., Des Jarlais, D. C., Friedman, S. R., Reid, T. R., & Bell, T. A. (1994). Risk of human immunodeficiency virus and hepatitis B virus in users of the Tacoma syringe exchange program, *Proceedings of the National Academy of Sciences Workshop on Needle Exchange and Bleach Distribution Programs*. National Academy Press, Washington, DC.

Hankins, C., Alary, M., Parent, R., Blanchette, C., Claessens, C., and the SurvUDI Working Group. (2002). Continuing HIV transmission among injection drug users in Eastern Central Canada: The SurvUDI Study, 1995–2000. *Journal of Acquired Immune Deficiency Syndrome* 30, pp. 514–521.

Heather, N., Wodak, A., Nadelmann, E., and O'Hare, P. (Eds.). (1993). *Psychoactive Drugs and Harm Reduction: From Faith to Science*. Whurr Publishers, London.

Heimer, R., and Singer, M. (2003). *Syringe Access, Use, and Discard—The I-91 Study*. Paper presented at the National Development and Research Institutes, New York.

Higgins, D. L., Galavotti, C., O'Reilly, K. R., Schnell, D. J., Moore, M., Rugg, D. L., and Johnson, R. (1991). Evidence for the effects of HIV antibody counseling and testing on risk behaviors. *Journal of the American Medical Association* 266, pp. 2419–2429.

Jackson, J., and Rotkiewicz, L. (1987). *A Coupon Program: AIDS Education and Drug Treatment*. Paper presented at the Third International Conference on AIDS, Washington, D.C.

Jacquez, J., Koopman, J., Simon, C., and Longini, I. (1994). Role of the primary infection in epidemic HIV infection of gay cohorts. *Journal of Acquired Immune Syndrome* 7, pp. 1169–1184.

Latkin, C. (1998). Outreach in natural settings: The use of peer leaders for HIV prevention among injection drug users' networks. *Public Health Reports* 113, pp. 151–159.

Latkin, C. A., Sherman, S., and Knowlton, A. (2003). HIV prevention among drug users: outcome of a network-oriented peer outreach intervention. *Health Psychology* 22(4), pp. 332–339.

Laumann, E., Gagnon, J. H., Michael, R., and Michaels, S. (1994). *The Social Organization of Sexuality: Sexual Practices in the United States*. University of Chicago Press, Chicago.

Mackay, J. L. (1994). The fight against tobacco in developing countries. *Tuberculosis and Lung Diseases* 75, pp. 8–24.

Manipur State AIDS Control Society. (2002). *HIV Sentinel Surveillance*. Impal, India: Manipur State AIDS Control Society.

Mann, J., Tarantola, J., and Netter, T. (1992). *AIDS in the World*. Harvard University, Cambridge, MA.

Maslow, C. B., Friedman, S. R., Perlis, T. E., Rockwell, R., and Des Jarlais, D. C. (2002). Changes in HIV seroprevalence and related behaviors among male injection drug users who do and do not have sex with men: New York City, 1990–1999. *American Journal of Public Health* 92(3), pp. 382–384.

Metzger, D., Woody, G., McLellan, A., O'Brien, C., Druley, P., Navaline, H., DePhilippis, D., Stolley, P., and Abrutyn, E. (1993). HIV seroconversion among IDUs in and out-of-treatment: An 18-month prospective follow-up. *AIDS* 6(9), pp. 1049–1056.

Nelson, K., Galai, N., Safaeian, M., Strathdee, S., Celentano, D., and Vlahov, D. (2002). Temporal trends in the incidence of human immunodeficiency virus infection and risk behavior among injection drug users in Baltimore, Maryland, 1988–1998. *American Journal of Epidemiology* 156(7), pp. 641–653.

National Institutes of Health. (1997). *Proceedings on the NIH Consensus Development Conference on Interventions to Prevent HIV Risk Behaviors.* Paper presented at the Proceedings on the NIH Consensus Development on Interventions to Prevent HIV Risk Behaviors, Bethesda, MD.

Normand, J., Vlahov, D., and Moses, L. E. (Eds.). (1995). *Preventing HIV Transmission: The Role of Sterile Needles and Bleach.* National Academy Press/National Research Council/Institute of Medicine, Washington, D.C.

O'Keefe, E., Kaplan, F., and Khoshnood, K. (1991). *Preliminary Report: City of New Haven Needle Exchange Program*: Office of Mayor John C. Daniels, New Haven, CT.

Ostrow, D. G. (1989). AIDS prevention through effective education. *Daedalus* 118, pp. 229–254.

Perez, K., Rodes, A., Merona, M., and Casabona, J. (2002). *Behavioural surveillance among intravenous drug users (IDUs) out-of-treatment in Barcelona (Spain), 1993–2000.* Paper presented at the Fourteenth International AIDS Conference, Barcelona, Spain.

Quan, V. M., Steketee, R. W., Valleroy, L., Weinstock, H., Karon, J., and Janssen, R. (2002). HIV incidence in the United States, 1978–1999. *Journal of Acquired Immune Deficiency Syndrome* 31, pp. 188–201.

Robertson, R. (Ed.). (1998). *Management of Drug Users in the Community: A Practical Handbook*, Oxford University Press Inc., New York.

Saidel, T. J., Des Jarlais, D. C., Peerapatanapokin, W., Dorabjee, J., Siddharth Singh, S., and Brown, T. (in press). Potential impact of HIV among IDUs on heterosexual transmission in Asian settings: The Asian epidemic model. *International Journal of Drug Policy*.

Selwyn, P., Feiner, C., Cox, C., Lipshutz, C., and Cohen, R. (1987). Knowledge about AIDS and high-risk behavior among intravenous drug abusers in New York City. *AIDS* 1, pp. 247–254.

Sherman, S. G., and Latkin, C. A. (2002). Drug users' involvement in the drug economy: implications for harm reduction and HIV prevention programs. *Journal of Urban Health* 79, pp. 266–277.

Spittal, P. M., Craib, K. J., Wood, E., Laliberte, N., Li, K., Tyndall, M. W., O'Shaughnessy, M. V., and Schechter, M. T. (2002). Risk factors for elevated HIV incidence rates among female injection drug users in Vancouver. *Canadian Medical Association Journal* 166(7), pp. 894–899.

Stimson, G. V. (1995). AIDS and injecting drug use in the United Kingdom, 1987–1993: the policy response and the prevention of the epidemic. *Social Science and Medicine* 41(5), pp. 699–716.

Stimson, G. V., Des Jarlais, D. C., and Ball, A. (Eds.). (1998). *Drug Injecting and HIV Infection: Global Dimensions and Local Responses.* UCL Press, London.

Stimson, G., Aceijas, C., Hickman, M., Dehne, K., and Rhodes, T. (2004). *Global Estimate of Injecting Drug Use.* Paper presented at the International Conference on the Reduction of Drug Use Related Harm, Melbourne, Australia.

Stolte, I. G., Dukers, N. H., de Wit, J. B., Fennema, J. S., and Coutinho, R. A. (2000). Increase in sexually transmitted infections among homosexual men in Amsterdam in relation to HAART. *Sex Transmitted Infections* 77, pp. 184–186.

Strathdee, S. A., van Ameijden, E. J. C., Mesquita, Wodak, A., Rana, S., and Vlahov, D. (1998). Can HIV epidemics among injection drug users be prevented? *AIDS* 12(suppl A), pp. 571–579.

Thompson, P. I., Jones, T. S., Cahill, K., and Medina, V. (1990). *Promoting HIV Prevention Outreach Activities Via Community-Based Organizations.* Paper presented at the Sixth International Conference on AIDS, San Francisco, CA.

UNAIDS/WHO. (2003). *AIDS Epidemic Update.* Joint United Nations Programme on HIV/AIDS (UNAIDS), Geneva.

van Ameijden, E., and Coutinho, R. (1998). Maximum impact of HIV prevention measures targeted at injecting drug users. *AIDS* 12(6), pp. 625–634.

Vanichseni, S., Des Jarlais, D. C., Choopanya, K., Friedmann, P., Wenston, J., Sonchai, W., Sotheran, J. L., Raktham, S., Carballo, M., and Friedman, S. R. (1993). Condom use with primary partners among injecting drug users in Bangkok, Thailand and New York City, United States. *AIDS* 7, pp. 887–891.

Vanichseni, S., Choopanya, K., Des Jarlais, D. C., Sakuntanaga, P., Kityaporn, D., Sujarita, S., Raktham, S., Hiranrus, K., Wasi, W., Mock, P. A., and Mastro, T. D. (2002). HIV among Injecting Drug Users in Bangkok: The First Decade. *International Journal of Drug Policy* 13, pp. 39–44.

Wiebel, W., Chene, D., & Johnson, W. (1990). *Adoption of Bleach Use in a Cohort of Street Intravenous Drug Users in Chicago.* Paper presented at the Sixth International Conference on AIDS, San Francisco, CA.

Wiebel, W. (1996). Ethnographic contributions to AID intervention strategies. In: Rhodes, T. and Hartnoll, R. (Eds.), *AIDS, Drugs and Prevention: Perspectives on Individual and Community Action,* Routledge, New York, pp. 186–200.

Wodak, A., and Lurie, P. (1996). A tale of two countries: Attempts to control HIV among injecting drug users in Australia and the United States. *Journal of Drug Issues* 27(1), pp. 117–134.

Wright, N., Vanichseni, S., Akarasewi, P., Wasi, C., and Choopanya, K. (1994). Was the 1988 HIV epidemic among Bangkok's injecting drug users a common source outbreak? *AIDS* 8, pp. 529–532.

D

Epidemiologic Information and Demand Reduction

14

Implications of Epidemiologic Information for Effective Drug Abuse Prevention Strategies

Zili Sloboda

1. INTRODUCTION

It has been only in the past two decades that drug abuse prevention researchers and practitioners in the United States have recognized the important contributions that epidemiologic study findings and methods have had on the development of

ZILI SLOBODA • Institute for Health and Social Policy, The University of Akron

211

effective preventive interventions. (Sloboda, 2003). These findings not only include what drugs are being used and in what ways but also the age at which most drug users initiate the use of illicit drugs and what characteristics and factors are most likely associated with increased risk to initiate drug use. It has been this information and advances in our understanding of behavior change that have had the most significant impact on the design of effective drug abuse preventive interventions. Epidemiology provides the knowledge to build prevention intervention strategies and to target interventions as well as providing the tools necessary to evaluate the impact of these interventions on the target population and, overtime, on the communities in which the target population lives.

This chapter discusses the relationship between epidemiologic and prevention intervention research in three sections. The first section will present a brief history of drug abuse prevention programming and research highlighting key landmarks of the progress of these fields. The second section will discuss the implications of epidemiologic findings for the design of prevention interventions and how epidemiologic methods are used for both needs assessments and outcome and impact evaluation studies. Finally, the last section will summarize what we have learned to date and identify key gaps in our knowledge base and suggest future directions for research and policy decisions.

2. PREVENTION PROGRAMMING AND RESEARCH

2.1. Defining Drug Abuse Prevention

Prevention of mental health and substance abuse problems in the United States is an evolving field. As late as the mid-1990s, new perspectives and conceptualization of the purposes of prevention had been discussed (Mrazek and Haggerty, 1994). Relinquishing the medical model of public health of primary, secondary and tertiary interventions, the field developed a new focus on a "spectrum" of interventions. In this spectrum, prevention interventions are implemented prior to the initial onset of a problem (Bukoski, 2003). Once a diagnostic status is achieved (using the DSM IV criteria), treatment interventions would apply. Efforts to assist with compliance to treatment regimens, to remain substance-free, and to be rehabilitated are considered "maintenance" interventions.

The purpose of substance abuse prevention programming in the United States is to delay the initiation of alcohol and tobacco use until the legal age and to reduce or eliminate the general use of these licit substances and of illicit substances including the misuse of solvents or other inhalants and prescription drugs. As the average age of initiation of drug use is between 13 and16, most prevention strategies target early adolescence. Over the past thirty years, the substance abuse prevention field has struggled to develop effective approaches to reach adolescents with messages that would influence them to make decisions not to use alcohol, tobacco, or illicit drugs. Most prevention programming in the early days focused on school-based curricula that included information dissemination, providing information about drugs and their effects; affective education, focusing on interpersonal growth and self-esteem with little attention to drugs and their effects; and, alternative approaches to substance use, providing recreational or community service activities to enhance self-reliance and to reduce feelings of alienation (Botvin and Griffin, 2003). However, it was not until the late 1970s and early 1980s that sufficient information on the epidemiology of substance use was available and that theories of human behavior were developed to form the foundations for the design and implementation of effective strategies.

2.2. Drug Abuse Prevention Research in the United States

With the establishment of the National Institute on Drug Abuse (NIDA) in 1974, the importance of drug abuse was recognized and its inclusion as one institute within the National Institutes of Health network in 1992 reinforced the noted association between drug abuse and health problems. Almost from the beginning, one of the major missions of NIDA was to create epidemiologic databases to achieve better estimates of the prevalence and incidence of drug abuse in the United States and to identify the determinants or risk factors that lead to drug use and abuse. These databases included population-based surveys such as the National Household Survey on Drug Abuse that targets persons aged 12 and older who reside in national representative samples of households (now under the auspices of the Substance Abuse and Mental Health Services Administration and renamed the National Survey on Drug Use and Health) and the Monitoring the Future Study (conducted under a grant by the University of Michigan) that since 1975 targeted 12th graders and since 1991, 8th and 10th graders, attending national representative samples of public and private schools. These surveys are cross-sectional and provide a "snap shot" of the prevalence and incidence of substance use. To complement these surveys, NIDA also supported longitudinal studies that would follow samples of adolescents over time to determine the factors associated with the onset of substance use. Bukoski (2003) identified these databases as landmark events for prevention as they have provided consistent findings relative to the origins and pathways of substance use. In their classic article, Hawkins and his associates (1992) have summarized the risk and protective factors that emerged from this research. This work was enhanced by Glantz and Pickens (1992) with the identification of those determinants that differentiate those among initiators of the use of drugs who become drug abusers or drug dependent.

The risk and protective factors approach to prevention had a great influence on the field and its reformulation of preventive and treatment interventions (Mrazek and Haggerty, 1994). With this information, three levels of prevention have been defined and embraced by drug abuse prevention researchers and practitioners. These levels address the varying degrees of risk found in the targeted population and are termed: universal, selective and indicated. Universal programs address general populations while selective programs target those segments of the population that present greater than normal risk to develop a disorder and indicated programs focus on those subgroups that exhibit signs or symptoms of developing a disorder. The recognition of the importance of theoretically derived models that specify the attitudes, perceptions and behaviors leading to substance use or other problem behaviors have become the target of prevention interventions (Coie et al., 1993).

The work of Richard Evans and his staff from the University of Houston (Evans, 1976; Evans et al., 1978) is cited as the origin of modern prevention. This group designed a smoking prevention program based on existing social and psychological factors and persuasive communications theory. The program was developed from research that showed that smoking was the result of social influences of peers and the media and that children could be inoculated against these pressures by making them aware of the rationales for these pressures and providing them the tools to resist these pressures and to practice their application. In addition, to address misconceptions students held about the prevalence of smoking among adolescents, periodic surveys were conducted among students on smoking behaviors with saliva sampling used to confirm these behaviors. These survey findings were shared with the students showing them that the actual rates of smoking were much lower than they estimated. The results of the evaluation of this program demonstrated that the students who participated in the program had significantly lower rates of initiating smoking than those in the control group. This was a major breakthrough in the substance abuse prevention field. Subsequent analyses of this work indicated that it was the feedback to the students that smoking was not a normative behavior that explained the findings (Botvin and Griffin, 2003).

Social learning theory that focuses on the interactions between people and their environments also served to shape approaches to prevention programs. The theory states that people learn new forms of behavior by seeing what others do and what the results or consequences are of those behaviors. The concept of self-efficacy expands social learning theory (Bandura, 1977) emphasizing the importance of an individual's belief in his/her competency to succeed in self-determined tasks or behaviors. Epidemiologic evidence indicates that most substance use among adolescents takes place through peer influence, therefore many substance use prevention programs incorporate the concept of self-efficacy, involve group activities, and often use peer models or assistants. These programs are designed (Botvin and Griffin, 2003) to increase students' resistance to those influences that encourage substance use, to focus on providing students with the skills they need to resist offers to use alcohol, tobacco or illicit drugs, and to give students opportunities to practice these resistance skills in virtual situations that are realistic to them.

NIDA has supported the evaluation of newly created substance use prevention programming through the 1980s until the present. The publication of the results of two NIDA-funded prevention studies in the prestigious Journal of the American Medical Association (Botvin et al., 1995; Pentz et al., 1989) gave the substance use prevention field new status in public health. The success of these and other programs led to another 'landmark' in the history of substance use prevention, the first NIDA-sponsored National Conference of Drug Abuse Prevention Research: Putting Research to Work for the Community in September 1996. The publication, Preventing Drug Use among Children and Adolescents: A Research-Based Guide (Sloboda and David, 1997) was a major outcome of the conference and has served as an important resource to prevention practitioners and policy makers. As Bukoski writes, "This publication clearly established the beginning of the evidence-based drug abuse prevention movement that has emerged across the country in the past 5 years." (Bukoski, 2003; p. 6) The Guide summarizes the findings from the research drawing consistent elements of effective prevention programming. This publication was the first of many other events that promoted evidence-based prevention programming. Since 1997, the United States Department of Education and the Center for Substance Abuse Prevention of the Substance Abuse and Mental Health Services Administration have both created processes through which the effectiveness of new prevention programs are reviewed for their inclusion on a list of promising or exemplary models.

3. LINKING EPIDEMIOLOGICAL INFORMATION TO PREVENTION

As indicated in the Introduction, there are two major roles that epidemiologic information serves for prevention. First is in the development of the intervention itself. Second is for conducting needs assessments for a community and to evaluate the outcomes and impact of the intervention.

3.1. Development of Prevention Interventions

In the 2003 edition of Preventing Drug Use among Children and Adolescents (NIDA, 2003), sixteen principles are listed that inform prevention development.

PRINCIPLES OF PREVENTION (NIDA, 2003)

1. **Prevention Programs should enhance protective factors and reverse or reduce risk factors.**

---

2. **Prevention Programs should address all forms of drug abuse, alone or in combination, including the underage use of legal drugs (e.g., tobacco or alcohol); the use of illegal drugs (e.g., marijuana or heroin); and the inappropriate use of legally obtained substances (e.g., inhalants), prescription medications, or over-the-counter drugs.**

3. **Prevention Programs should address the type of drug abuse problem in the local community, target modifiable risk factors, and strengthen identified protective factors.**

4. **Prevention Programs should be tailored to address risks specific to population or audience characteristics, such as age, gender, and ethnicity, to improve program effectiveness.**

5. **Family-based prevention programs should enhance family bonding and relationships and include parenting skills; practice in developing, discussing, and enforcing family policies on substance abuse; and training in drug education and information.**

6. **School programs can be designed to intervene as early as preschool to address risk factors for drug abuse, such as aggressive behavior, poor social skills, and academic difficulties.**

7. **Elementary school programs should target improving academic and social-emotional learning to address risk factors for drug abuse, such as early aggression, academic failure, and school dropout focusing on self-control, emotional awareness, communication, social problem-solving, and academic support.**

8. **Middle or junior high and high school programs should increase academic and social competence focusing on academic support, communication, peer relationships, self-efficacy and assertiveness, drug resistance skills, reinforcement of anti-drug attitudes, and strengthening of personal commitments against drug abuse.**

9. **General population programs should address key transition points, such as the transition to middle school.**

10. Community programs that combine two or more effective programs, such as family-based and school-based programs, can be more effective than a single program alone.

11. Community programs reaching populations in multiple settings—for example, schools, clubs, faith-based organizations, and the media—are most effective when they present consistent, community-wide messages in each setting.

12. When communities adapt a program for their specific needs they should retain core elements of the original research-based intervention.

13. **Programs should be long-term with repeated interventions to reinforce the original prevention goals.**

14. Programs should include instructors trained in good class-room management practices.
15. Programs are most effective when they employ interactive techniques that allow for active involvement in learning about drug abuse and reinforcing skills.
16. Programs can be cost-effective.

Ten of the 16 principles (in bold in the table) reflect information derived from epidemiologic studies. The information is derived from both descriptive and analytic studies (see Chapter 1) such as age of onset, sequencing patterns of substance use, and risk and protective factors associated with the initiation of substance use. The following discusses the epidemiologic evidence on each of these issues.

3.1.1. Age of Onset

Before discussing the age of onset or initiation of substance use, it is important to have a picture of the extent of drug use in the general population. Briefly, according to the most recent National Survey on Drug Use and Health report (2002) an estimated 19.5 million people aged 12 and older used at least one illicit drug in the month prior to survey. Almost 60 percent of these drug users used only marijuana while an additional 20 percent used marijuana and at least one other drug and another 20 percent used an illicit drug(s) other than marijuana. The information on the prevalence of drug use by age group showed that for three decades the rates of drug use were higher for those aged 18 through 25 than any other age group and that reports of new drug use are highest among teenagers. Information from the Monitoring the Future Survey (MTF) shows that the percentage of teen use of tobacco, alcohol and illicit drugs increases between 150 percent and 200 percent when students move from the 8th to the 10th grade. Clearly, substance use, particularly illicit drug use, is a problem of our youth. Most cross-sectional and prospective studies show that the average age of onset is under age 18 years and generally between 13 and 16. (OAS, 2004).

Patterns of drug use by youth have varied over time. Both the NHSDA (now NSDUH) and MTF have shown that overall drug use among adolescents had peaked in the late 1970s with downturns noted during the 1980s and then short-term increases in the early 1990s. Although marijuana has been the drug of choice through all of these periods, each decade has seen other drugs being used. The late 1970s through the 1980s showed increased use of cocaine while more recent surveys show upsurges in the initiation of drugs such as ecstasy (MDMA), LSD, PCP, and the misuse of prescription drugs. The most interesting observation from MTF is the downward trends in cigarette use peaking among high school seniors in 1977 when the estimated lifetime prevalence of use was 75.7 percent and then declining to a low of 53.7 percent in 2003 (MTF, 2004). Explanations for these up and down trends have been linked to attitudes about the consequences associated with the use of specific drugs and to perceptions as to the level of general social tolerance for drug use. This is particularly noteworthy for cigarette use as well as for marijuana and cocaine use (Bachman et al., 1990; Bachman et al., 1998).

3.1.2.   The Sequencing of Substance Use

A controversial issue in the field of drug abuse epidemiology is the "gateway" theory that explains the initiation of illicit drugs or the sequencing pattern of drug use. The concept was introduced to the field by Denise Kandel in 1975 and in principle states that individuals progress along a specific pathway from alcohol and/or tobacco use to the use of marijuana and from the use of marijuana to the use of other illicit drugs (Kandel et al., 1992). Several other prospective studies of youngsters have had similar findings. Whether there is a physiological or social mechanism at play that explains this pattern of substance use is unclear. What it seems to signify is that one's risk to move on to marijuana is **much** higher than if one never smoked or drank and the risk of moving on to cocaine is **much** higher for someone who ever used marijuana than for someone who never did. It is the lack of a clear mechanism that brings the theory into question. However, the epidemiologic evidence is so consistent that prevention specialists have incorporated the concept of progression into their programs and address the use of tobacco and alcohol as well other drugs relevant to the age group represented in their target groups. (Scheirer et al., 2001)

3.1.3.   Risk and Protection

Until the mid-1970s most of our understanding of the determinants of the initiation of the use of alcohol, tobacco or other drugs by children and adolescents came from cross-sectional studies of adolescent or adult substance users. The nature of these studies could not support causal relationships. With the establishment of a number of longitudinal studies by NIDA that followed children through their teenage years into adulthood it was possible to identify not only those factors that put children at risk of drug use and abuse but also for those children most at risk for using drugs, those factors that protected them from being involved in drug use. Using the findings from both the cross-sectional and prospective studies, several drug abuse epidemiologists have attempted to categorize risk and protective factors (Hawkins et al., 1992; Flay and Petraitis, 2003, Brook et al., 1988, 2003; Newcomb and Felix-Ortiz, 1992; Pandina, 1998). In general, these groupings include personal, family, peer, and environmental determinants. Many of these factors are both direct and indirect contributors to drug using behaviors. Sorting the potential effects of any or all of these factors has become a great challenge to the prevention field (Flay and Petraitis, 2003). The difficulty has been in attributing degree or level of risk associated with these factors across the developmental periods of a child's life.

By taking the developmental approach, it then becomes clear that at various key social and psychological stages of growth, some of these factors may be more important than others. For example, parents and primary caregivers serve an essential role in providing nurturing, stimulation and modeling to enable infants to bond with other humans and to communicate with the world around them. Failure to form these warm attachments has been linked to a number of problems in subsequent phases such as poor language skills and cognitive ability as well as to inappropriate self-regulatory behavior in early childhood and later, drug abuse. (McCartney et al., 2004).

Research focusing on protective factors supports this perspective (Brook et al., 1990). Investigations of groups of children determined to be susceptible to drug use but who do not become involved with drugs, have found that early attachments to an adult can serve to protect children from initiating the use of drugs. What is yet unclear from this research, however, is the weight these protective factors need to carry to overcome risk. For instance, would having a strong teacher role model counter failure to bond within the early family?

Other research examines the processes that are closer or more proximate to becoming a drug user such as the availability of drugs, knowledge on how to obtain drugs, as well as having more positive attitudes about drugs. For example, research has found that when children understand the negative physical, psychological, and social effects of drugs and when they perceive social disapproval of drug use by their friends and families, they tend to avoid drug initiation (Bachman et al., 1990; Bachman et al., 1998).

More recent studies address the question of progression from use to abuse or dependence on drugs. A significant work that stimulated the thinking in this area was the book, Vulnerability to Drug Abuse (Glantz and Pickens, 1992) that includes papers from a conference held by NIDA in 1989 entitled, Transition from Drug Use to Abuse/Dependence. Glantz and Pickens summarized the findings of this research, differentiating factors associated with drug use from those associated with drug abuse. They point out that although drug use tends to be more related to social and peer factors, drug abuse has more biological or psychological precursors. (p. 9)

Most prevention programs today either address one of more of these risk factors or provide reinforcement to existing protective. (For examples, see NIDA, 2003).

3.2. Needs Assessments and Program Evaluation

Planning prevention programming for communities generally requires an assessment of the extent and nature of the substance abuse problem (Brown, 1997). Studies that compare substance use problems at the community level show that there is often wide-variation in the types of substances used, in the characteristics of the user population, and in the factors that may be most associated with the initiation and maintenance of substance use. With the greater availability of and pressure to use effective prevention programs, more and more communities are struggling to determine which best meets the needs of their communities. Several planners and researchers have developed planning models that are becoming more widely used by community coalitions, partnerships, and planning boards (e.g., Hawkins et al., 1992; SAMHSA, 2002). Most of these models use a logic system or step-by-step strategic planning approach. In general these steps include conducting a needs assessment and an inventory of available social and physical capital (skills, competencies, and resources), setting priorities among the identified needs, selecting strategies to address these needs, implementing the strategies, and evaluation. Epidemiological methods serve to conduct the needs assessments and to conduct evaluations, particularly when community-wide strategies are used. Several of these methods are discussed in more detail in other chapters of this book. Brown (1997) and others (Hawkins et al., 1992) suggest the use of archival and survey information to establish need. Generally multiple methods are encouraged. Clearly, before any assessments are initiated, it is important for planners first to decide what they want to target. This sounds like a chicken and egg dilemma, however, if the concern is to prevent adolescents at high risk of substance use from becoming drug abusers, other methods may be employed. These may include random drug testing or the use of an assessment instrument such as the Drug Use Screening Inventory (DUSI) (Tarter et al., 1992) or the Problem Oriented Screening Instrument for Teenagers (POSIT) (McLaney et al., 1994).

Archival information provides a snapshot of current drug abuse patterns within the community and if built into ongoing surveillance systems, has the potential of identifying new patterns that should be addressed in prevention strategies that include broad community involvement of law enforcement, the media, the schools, families, faith-based organizations, and local government and businesses. Archival data for juveniles such as school drop out rates or academic standings, child abuse, arrest patterns, and census data help identify geographic patterns of need.

School surveys should be conducted not only with students who are within the "at risk" age group but also with younger students to determine risk status, existing perceptions and attitudes of substance use, intentions to use tobacco, alcohol or other drugs, and actual use. Conducting school surveys on a routine basis, either annually or bi-annually, will help identify new problem areas and to assess the overall impact of prevention strategies. The tools for such needs assessments and evaluations are derived from the field of epidemiology and are discussed in the chapters by Sloboda et al. and Adlaf.

Drug testing as a prevention tool remains somewhat controversial in the United States yet is strongly advocated by the Office for National Drug Control Policy. The controversy surrounding drug testing is two-pronged. The first issue is whether random drug testing impinges on the rights of adolescents and their parents. The second issue relates to how it is best used within a prevention framework. The outcomes of both drug testing and the use of such instruments as the DUSI and POSIT can be used to identify individuals or can be aggregated for a school or other group setting. Because of the problem of labeling the individual or group, it is important to view these approaches as archival records and surveys as tools of prevention planning.

Just as these data collection approaches are helpful in making an assessment of community needs these also serve as excellent evaluation tools. Communities may consider the needs assessment phase of planning as establishing a baseline prior to implementation of an intervention. Part of the implementation plan should be an evaluation that sets periodic markers that assess progress toward meeting short-, intermediate- and long-term objectives.

4. CONCLUSIONS

Clearly, over the past two to three decades there has been an accumulation of knowledge about the epidemiology and the prevention of drug abuse. However many questions remain unanswered that impede further progress in the prevention of drug abuse. Since the mid 1970s data systems have allowed the monitoring of increases and decreases in the use of illicit substances. However, only crude explanations are available as to why these trends occur. Not only are explanations lacking to explain these up and down trends, but we do not fully understand differential and changing patterns of drug use. For instance, reports from the Community Epidemiology Work Group that is supported by NIDA indicate that drug abuse patterns are defined by time and space. Some patterns are national in scope such as the use of marijuana, heroin and cocaine while others are regional such as the use of methamphetamine and PCP. Some patterns of drug use are long-term (e.g., injecting heroin) while others last but a few years (e.g., L.S.D.).

Furthermore, much of the behavior we call "drug abuse" and its associated etiology is based on the findings from cross-sectional and longitudinal studies. However, the factors implicated with drug abuse are but indicators of a number of complicated underlying processes. The need to develop a set of socio-bio-psychological theories of drug abuse is evident to guide future epidemiologic studies. Such theories must reflect the phased nature of drug abuse behaviors (from initiation through dependency), the interaction of the individual within various social groups and society, and the changing nature of drug abuse within the context of societal structures and processes, norms, values, and interests. Such a theoretical perspective would enable the strategic targeting of preventive interventions.

Finally, and perhaps most provocative, is our failure to understand why the use of illicit drugs among young people is increasing in most countries around the world. Boundaries between countries and cultures are becoming more porous, easing the transport of drugs. The commonality of patterns of drug use however does not imply that there is a commonality of prevention strategies. More cross-national and cross-cultural studies of these strategies are needed to further the understanding of what aspects of these interventions are the most effective.

We are entering the 21st Century with great challenges ahead. Yet, those who began addressing these issues over three decades ago have provided us the concepts and the tools to advance our understanding of drug abuse in order to halt its devastating impact on individuals, on their families, and on society.

REFERENCES

Bachman, J.G., Johnston, L.D. & O'Malley, P.M. (1990). Explaining the recent decline in cocaine use among young adults: further evidence that perceived risks and disapproval lead to reduced drug use. *Journal of Health and Social Behavior* 31(2), pp. 173–184.

Bachman, J.G., Johnston, L.D. & O'Malley, P.M. (1998). Explaining recent increases in students' marijuana use: impacts of perceived risks and disapproval, 1976 through 1996. *American Journal of Public Health* 88(6), pp. 887–892.

Bandura, A. (1977). *Social Learning Theory*. Prentice-Hall, Englewood Cliffs, NJ.

Botvin, G.J., Baker, E., Dusenbury, L., Tortu, S., & Botvin, E.M. (1995). Long-term follow-up results of a randomized drug abuse prevention trial in a White middle-class population. *Journal of the American Medical Association* 273(14), pp. 1106–1112.

Brook, J.S., Brook, D.W., Richter, L. & Whiteman, M. (2003). Risk and protective factors of adolescent drug use: implications for prevention programs. In: Sloboda, Z. & Bukoski, W.J. (Eds.), *Handbook of Drug Abuse Prevention: Theory, Science, and Practice*. Kluwer Academic/Plenum Publishers, New York.

Botvin, G.J. & Griffin, K.W. (2003). Drug abuse prevention curricula in schools. In: Sloboda, Z. & Bukoski, W.J. (Eds.), *Handbook of Drug Abuse Prevention: Theory, Science, and Practice*. Kluwer Academic/Plenum Publishers, New York.

Brown, B.S. (1997). Drug abuse prevention needs assessment methodologies: a review of the literature. NIDA Resource Center for Health Services Research. http://www.nida.nih.gov/about/organization/DESPR/HSR/da-pre/Brownprevention.htm.

Bukoski, W.J. (2003). The emerging science of drug abuse prevention. In: Sloboda, Z. & Bukoski, W.J. (Eds.), *Handbook of Drug Abuse Prevention: Theory, Science, and Practice*. Kluwer Academic/Plenum Publishers, New York.

Coie, J.D., Watt, N.F., West, S.G., Hawkins, J.D., Asarnow, J.R., Markman, H.J., Ramey, S.L., Shure, M.B., & Long, B. (1993). The science of prevention: a conceptual framework and some directions for a national research program. *American Psychologist* 48(10), pp. 1013–1022.

Evans, R. I. (1976). Smoking in children: developing a social psychological strategy of deterrence. *Preventive Medicine* 5, pp. 122–127.

Evans, R.I., Rozelle, R.M., Mittlemark, M.B., Hansen, W.B., Bane, A.L. & Havis, J. (1978). Deterring the onset of smoking in children: knowledge of immediate physiological effects and coping with peer pressure, media pressure, and parent modeling. *Journal of Applied Social Psychology* 8, pp. 126–135.

Flay, B.R. & Petraitis, H. (2003). Bridging the gap between substance use prevention theory and practice. In: Sloboda, Z. & Bukoski, W.J. (Eds.), *Handbook of Drug Abuse Prevention: Theory, Science, and Practice*. Kluwer Academic/Plenum Publishers, New York.

Glantz, M.D. & Pickens, R.W. (1992). Vulnerability to drug abuse: introduction and overview. In: Glantz, M.D. & Pickens, R.W. (Eds.), *Vulnerability to Drug Abuse*. American Psychological Association, Washington, D.C., pp. 1–14.

Hawkins, J.D., Catalano, R.F. & Associates. (1992). *Communities That Care*. Jossey-Bass Publishers, San Francisco, CA.

Hawkins, J.D., Catalano, R.F. & Miller, J.Y. (1992). Risk and protective factors for alcohol and other drug problems in adolescence and early adulthood: implications for substance abuse prevention. *Psychological Bulletin* 112(1), pp. 64–105.

Kandel, D.B. (1975). Stages in adolescent involvement in drug use. *Science*, 190(4217), 912–914.

Kandel, D.B., Yamaguchi, K. & Chen, K. (1992). Stages of progression in drug involvement from adolescence to adulthood: further evidence for the gateway theory. *Journal of Studies of Alcohol* 53(5), pp. 447–457.

Mzarek, P. J. & Haggerty, R.J. (1994). *Reducing Risks for Mental Disorders*. National Academy Press, Washington, D.C.

McCartney, K., Owen, M.T., Booth, C.L., Clarke-Stewart, A. & Vandell, D.L. (2004). Testing a maternal attachment model of behavior problems in early childhood. *Journal of Child Psychology and Psychiatry* 45(4), pp. 765–778.

McLaney, M.A., Del Boca, F.K. & Babor, T. (1994). A validation study of the Problem Oriented Screening Instrument for Teenagers (POSIT). *Journal of Mental Health* 3, pp. 363–376.

National Institute on Drug Abuse. (2003). *Preventing Drug Abuse among Children and Adolescents: A Research-Based Guide*. NIH Publication No. 04–4212(B).

Newcomb, M. D. & Felix-Ortiz, M. (1992). Multiple protective and risk factors for drug use and abuse: cross-sectional and prospective findings. *Journal of Personality and Social Psychology* 63, pp. 280–296.

Office of Applied Studies (2004). *2002 National Survey on Drug Use and Health*, http://www.oas.samhsa.gov/NHSDA/2k2NSDUH/Results/2k2results.htm#chap6.

Pandina, R.J. (1998). Risk and protective factor models in adolescent drug use: Putting them to work for prevention. *National Conference on Drug Abuse Prevention Research: Presentations, Papers, and Recommendations* (pp. 17–26). NIH Publication No. 98–4293.

Pentz, M.A., Dwyer, J.H., MacKinnon, D.P., Flay, B.R., Hansen, W.B., Wang, E.Y. & Johnson, C.A. (1989). A multi-community trial for primary prevention of adolescent drug abuse: effects on drug use prevalence. *Journal of the American Medical Association* 261, pp. 3259–3266.

Scheier, L.M., Botvin, G.J. & Griffin, K.W. (2001). Preventive intervention effects on developmental progression in drug use: structural equation modeling analyses using longitudinal data. *Prevention Science* 2(2), pp. 91–112.

Sloboda, Z. & David, S.L. (1997). *Preventing Drug Abuse among Children and Adolescents: A Research-Based Guide*. NIH Publication No. 97–4212.

Substance Abuse and Mental Health Services Administration. (2002). Achieving Outcomes: A Practitioner's Guide to Effective Prevention. http://www.modelprograms.samhsa.gov/pdfs/Achieving Outcomes.pdf.

Tarter, R.E., Laird, S.B., Bukstein,O. & Kaminer, Y. (1992). Validation of the Adolescent Drug Use Screening Inventory: preliminary findings. *Psychology of Addictive Behaviors* 6(4), pp. 233–236.

15

The Role of Treatment Data in Studying the Epidemiology of Substance Use and Abuse

Robert L. Hubbard

1. INTRODUCTION

The most complete and informative data on substance abuse can be available from the population that has the most involvement with substance abuse. This population can be found most efficiently in the substance abusers treated. The data from treated substance abusers offers detailed information on the dysfunctional patterns of substance abuse and on the types of drugs creating the most problems. The major challenge in using information from treated populations is its application to the more global estimation of the nature of the substance abuse problem and trends in the patterns of substance abuse. This chapter has four sections. The first

ROBERT L. HUBBARD • Center for Community-Based Studies, National Development and Research Institutes provides a framework of how data from treated substance abusers can fit into an overall epidemiological framework. The second section will review the epidemiology of substance use within treatment populations followed by a discussion on how data from treated populations has been used in epidemiological estimation. Finally, recommendations are made as to how information on treated populations can be made more useful for general epidemiological perspectives.

2.   A CONCEPTUAL FRAMEWORK

Information on individuals treated for substance abuse can provide the most detailed and comprehensive data on substance abuse patterns. The patterns of multiple substance use can be studied in combination with overall level of impairment. The critical question is how this information can be used in a general epidemiological model.

As described in other chapters the total epidemiology of substance abuse must encompass multiple but temporally separate domains of the population: households, institutions and those without a permanent residence. At any one time the treated population is more likely to be in the latter two domains. For example the 2002 national data on treatment admissions shows that 22.9 percent of the treated population were living in a supervised setting and 12.6 percent are identified as homeless (TEDS, 2002). Despite this fact, in a given year, a high proportion of the substance abusing population does reside in a household at some time, but most have been in institutions at some time in their lives.

The first study that attempted to delineate the overlap and independence of the multiple populations was the Washington D.C. Metropolitan Area Drug Study (Research Triangle Institute, 1994). The study populations for this research included arrestees, homeless, pregnant, school, and household populations in addition to a sample from treatment programs. Almost nine of every ten clients in methadone, residential, or inpatient treatment had been in an institution at some time in their lives and over half had been in institutions in the past year. About half of residential clients, a fifth of methadone clients, and a tenth of inpatient clients had been incarcerated in the past year. About one in ten clients reported being without a permanent residence in the past year. About 90 percent of women entering treatment had been pregnant and about 10 percent were pregnant in the past year. About 50 percent of methadone clients had dropped out of high school and a third of inpatient clients had dropped out of high school. Compared to the general household population the clinic populations in methadone tended to be more male (63 versus 48 percent), more African American (75 versus 27 percent), single (50 versus 33 percent), less likely to complete high school (42 versus 13 percent) and not to be employed full time (70 percent versus 35 percent). The inpatient population profile is somewhat closer to the household population in age, employment and marital status, but more similar to the methadone population in gender and education level.

The results of this comparison suggest the need for careful consideration of the use of "treatment" samples in the inference of general epidemiological estimates or trends. Clearly there are major differences among the types of drug users entering different types of treatment programs and clear differences with the household and school populations used to develop estimates and trends. The following discussions will attempt to keep these important differences in mind and suggest how to take the complexity of the treatment population into account in a general epidemiological model.

3. TREATMENT POPULATIONS

Three main types of data show how treatment populations can be used to provide epidemiological data. The first is the rich database established in three major national research studies of treatment from the late sixties to the early nineties. The second is the national data base initially developed as the Client Oriented Data Acquisition Process (CODAP) which has been resurrected as the Treatment Episode Data Set (TEDS) in 1992. The final source is the set of monitoring systems being developed by States which were stimulated by the Center for Substance Abuse Treatment (CSAT) TOPPS grants in the mid 1990s.

The three research studies are the Drug Abuse Reporting Program (DARP) collecting over 44,000 admission records from 52 federally supported community agencies from 1969–1973, the Treatment Outcome Prospective Study (TOPS) conducted between 1979 and 1981 with 11,750 clients in 41 community treatment programs, and the Drug Abuse Treatment Outcome Study (DATOS) from 1991–1993 with 10,010 clients in 96 programs. The research attempted to maintain the comparability of questions and to the extent possible the same communities and programs. Comparisons among these data bases were examined by Craddock and colleagues (1997). The most striking result was the change in drug use pattern across all treatment modalities. In the late sixties, 28 percent of clients reported using heroin with few if any other drugs. In the late 1970s, use of multiple drugs with alcohol was the modal pattern, with only one in 50 clients reporting using heroin only. It is also important to note that less than one percent of clients in the late sixties or seventies reported using cocaine only and only about one fourth of clients reported cocaine use at least once a week. This pattern changed drastically by the early 1990s with the prominence of cocaine. Reports of weekly or more frequent use doubled from the late seventies while reports of heroin and multiple use patterns decreased. In the 1990s, clients tended to be older, better educated, less employed, and more dependent on public assistance. With the emergence of problems of infectious diseases, especially AIDS, the population appears to have presented with more complexities requiring comprehensive treatment. To enable further investigation of many of these issues, the data from TOPS and DATOS has been made available on public use files.

From 1976 to 1981, the CODAP provided basic information on client demographics, prior treatment, drug use, and employment for all clients in programs receiving federal funding. The data for approximately 250,000 clients provided both state level data as well as trend data. One major use of the CODAP data was the comparison with data bases such as TOPS to determine the potential generalizability of research studies to the national population of clients. The comparison of TOPS and CODAP data revealed consistent patterns of demographic characteristics both across modalities as well as over time. The major discrepancies occurred in the identification of primary drugs of abuse and more complex patterns of use. CODAP was limited to the report of primary, secondary and tertiary drugs of abuse, while the description of complex patterns of multiple drug use in TOPS often involved a minimum of heroin, cocaine, marijuana and alcohol. A second issue involved the clinical assignment of a primary drug by a counselor in CODAP compared to the self-report of a problem by clients in TOPS. The rates of reported primary drug problem usually differed by less than 5 percent (81 percent heroin in methadone programs in CODAP compared to 77 percent in TOPS). A third issue was the self-report of having no problems with drugs by about one of every seven clients, particularly those referred from the criminal justice system. The value of the CODAP data was the opportunity to look at state differences and examine basic trends over time. Unfortunately, the system became voluntary in the early 1980s and the data became much less useful.

In the late 1980s the utility of complete and comprehensive data on treatment admissions received renewed support. The Treatment Episode Data Set (TEDS) was designed to again track admissions for all clients receiving federal funding. A data base was established in the Substance Abuse and Mental Health Data Archive (SAMHDA) at the University of Michigan http://www.icpsr.umich .edu/SAMHDA. Over 80 studies had used the data base through 2003 (The DASIS Report, May 30, 2003).

One report (The Treatment Episode Data Set April 1, 2002) examined trends on five issues; primary drug of abuse, co-abuse of alcohol and drugs, admission rates by state, demographic characteristics, and socioeconomic status. The results showed a decrease from 1992 to 2000 in reports of alcohol as the primary problem (59 percent in 1992 to 45 percent in 2000). Reports of primary opioid use increased from 12 percent in 1992 to 17 percent in 2000. This increase was accompanied by a corresponding decrease from 18 percent to 14 percent in reports of cocaine as the primary drug. Reports of marijuana as the primary drug increased by a factor of 2.5 from 6 percent in 1992 to 15 percent in 2000. While the report recognized the co-abuse of alcohol and other drugs by almost half the admissions (42 percent), the TEDS assessment of drug use is still limited to primary, secondary, and tertiary drugs used.

An extensive analysis of reports of primary drug use was also made available by state. Although states varied in the levels of reports of different primary drugs at admission, a number of interesting and consistent trends were noted across states. Declines in reports of alcohol as the primary drug of abuse were replicated across a number of states. Eighteen states reported increases of over 100 percent for admissions for heroin use. The decline in cocaine reports was also consistent across states. The reports of use of methamphetamine increased from 1992 to 2000 and showed a pattern of moving from west to east. While the data are interesting, a number of key questions are raised that might usefully be addressed. A multivariate trend analysis might indicate possible population or ecological characteristics that influence trends or levels of use. The extensive descriptive data reported begs for a more systematic, theory based analysis. The results of such analyses may enable epidemiologists and treatment administrators to better predict future trends and prepare to address new patterns of abuse or related problems.

Trends in demographic characteristics may provide a framework for more systematic analysis. The demographic trends showed stability in the proportion of males and in the racial/ethnic composition of the treatment population. A decline in the proportion of young adults aged 25–34 from 40 percent in 1992 to 27 percent in 2000 may suggest some hypotheses for the changes in reports of drugs used. The hypothesis would be that usage patterns differ by age group, therefore accounting for the trends. Other socioeconomic characteristics (employment and education) were interpreted as showing a much more disadvantaged population entering treatment compared to national averages. These levels of socioeconomic status did not change over time and state variations were not addressed.

Another report (The DASIS Report April 9, 2004) looked at the number of admissions with psychiatric disorders accompanying substance abuse. The data base was over 600,000 annual admissions in twenty states from 1995–2001. Reports of co-occurring disorders increased from 12 percent to 16 percent over the six years. The reports of co-occurring disorders were associated with alcohol as the primary drug (45 percent compared to 38 percent) and gender (44 percent for females compared to 30 percent for males). The reports of co-occurring disorders were also positively related to the residential/rehabilitative service setting and self-referral to treatment. Again the descriptive analysis raises more questions that need to be addressed by more detailed analyses over time and within and across states.

·The brief overview of two major types of data bases, both in the public domain demonstrate that treatment data by itself offers interesting and important contributions to epidemiological investigation. There are clear differences across and within states and a number of important trends have been identified. The major gap is a comprehensive, theoretically based investigation of the epidemiology of treatment admissions, particularly in terms of patterns of drug abuse and key co-occurring disorders. In addition to providing scientific contributions to the field of epidemiology, the findings can also help to guide policy and practice to meet a constantly changing client population with many serious problems. To support

these analyses the data from state monitoring systems can be better incorporated
into the design and analysis of epidemiological investigations. While most are
based on the core TEDS items, many states have expanded their data base to
include the Addiction Severity Index and other data elements.

4.   INTEGRATION WITH OTHER DATA SOURCES

Treatment data have proven valuable in use with other data sources. Three
main areas of exploration have utilized treatment data. The first is the use of
treatment data as one of multiple sources of data used to assess drug use patterns
across populations, geographic areas and over time. The second is the systematic
inclusion of information about treatment in samples from more general populations
to make prevalence estimates for the population. The third approach is to use
treatment data in statistical models to predict usage patterns, trends and prevalence.

In 1974, a pioneering effort was launched to try to better understand the epidemiology of substance abuse with a unique perspective. Data was to be collected
from multiple sources and reviewed periodically by experts from different disci-
plines knowledgeable about drug use in different communities (NIDA, 1998). This
network became known as the Community Epidemiology Work Group. The group
considered treatment information in combination with survey data, law enforcement data, hospital sources such as emergency room admissions, public health
information including infectious diseases such as HIV/AIDS and hepatitis, school
system data, vital statistics including alcohol and drug related deaths, and other
community data sources. The utility of the other data sources is discussed elsewhere in this book. The unique role and the potential problems of using treatment
data in this context are important to understand.

While providing very useful information on drug use patterns historically
and ecologically, the relationship of treatment data to the other sources is not well
understood. It is also likely that the relationship will differ across communities and
over time. As Kozel and Sloboda point out (NIDA, 1998), treatment admissions do
not represent the total population of users. Second, the pattern of use presented at
the time of admission to treatment has likely taken significant time to develop and
worsen. Thus, inferences for new users may be limited. Ecologically, the treatment
system functions in a health care and criminal justice environment that is likely
to change over time and differ across communities. Thus, the clients entering the
treatment system may change depending on the priorities and practices of the larger
community context. This final issue is an important focus for and emerging area of
organizational research on treatment systems. The relationship of organizational
change and the epidemiology of treatment admissions is still poorly understood.

Once the limitations of the data are understood, a more vexing problem is
presented. In many cases the various data sources do not provide the same picture

either in terms of trends, population estimates, or ecological comparisons. The annual CEWG reports (National Institute on Drug Abuse, 1996; 1997) often provide and cite these differences. The challenge then is making sense of the multiple pictures and understanding how and why the data sources may reveal accurate, but fragmented pictures of the overall drug abuse problem. The unique contribution of the CEWG is the reasonable attempt to create a mosaic from the fragments to better inform science, policy, and practice.

The second major advance in the field is the attempt to capture cross population data in different types of studies. The first to attempt this was the previously mentioned District of Columbia Metropolitan Area Drug Study (DCMADS). Subsequent to that study which asked similar questions about treatment participation across various population samples, the approach was adopted for the National Survey on Drug Use and Health (NSDUH) formerly known up to 2001 as the National Household Survey on Drug Abuse (NHSDA). In all surveys, questions are asked on dependence and abuse. In addition, questions are asked on the need for treatment for alcohol and illicit drug problems as well as serious mental illness. For the first time it is now possible to obtain estimates of treatment need using a population-based model not only at the national, but also at the state level. The 2002 results (Office of Applied Studies, 2004) showed that in the past year approximately 8 percent of the population 12 and older had alcohol dependence or abuse and 3 percent had dependence or abuse of illicit drugs. The rates for alcohol abuse or dependence across states varied from 6 percent to 10 percent. The rates for drug abuse or dependence ranged from 2 percent to 4 percent. These percentages translate into almost 15 million persons abusing or dependent on alcohol, 4 million abusing or dependent on drugs only, and another 3 million abusing or dependent on both.

Unfortunately, even with the large scale of the study and the large numbers of persons estimated to have problems, the number of persons in the sample who report receiving treatment is too small to provide stable statistical estimates. The calculations that are based on acceptable data indicate that 7.3 percent of the household population over age 12 needed but did not receive treatment for alcohol problems and 2.7 percent of the household population needed but did not receive treatment for drug problems; estimates and numbers not much different than the rates of abuse and dependence. Using population data and a number of key covariates to support statistical modeling, it was possible to project the unmet treatment need for all states and the District of Columbia.

Similar approaches to statistical modeling have been used to estimate the numbers of different types of comparatively rare types of users, such as heroin addicts. Brodsky (1985) delineated these methods as mathematical models and dynamic simulation. The initial mathematical model is based on a technique known as capture-recapture. In this the application of this technique first by Greenwood (1971) and then by Woodward, Bonett and Brecht (1985), the admission and readmission to treatment is a key element. In their application, Woodward et al., used the previously mentioned CODAP data. While the level of statistical error was substantial, the authors did feel that acceptable inferences of trends could be made given sufficiently large samples.

A more general model attempting to estimate the number of users was the Persistent Poppy developed by Levin, Roberts and Hirsch (1975). Using a complex series of equations it is theoretically possible to develop estimates to simulate usage patterns as well as the need for treatment. Gardiner and Shreckengost (1985) applied similar technology to estimating the amount of heroin imports. Unfortunately, the robustness of the available data has not supported stable estimates from these models. Both models depend largely on the relationship of use to admission to treatment; a relationship we have not been able to understand or model to the level required for complex estimation techniques.

5. CONCLUSION

In this chapter a number of uses of treatment data to support epidemiological research, analysis, and interpretation were reviewed. It is clear that treatment data alone or integrated with other sources of information can provide important insights into the epidemiology of drug abuse. The major contributions appear to be in estimating trends and comparing these across geographic or demographic groups. The utility of treatment data to accurately estimate prevalence is limited by the proportionately few persons who enter treatment.

Despite these limitations, much more can and should be done to better utilize the rich information from treatment data bases. The first is to reach consensus on key questions on usage patterns, institutional contact (e.g. jails, social service, health care, etc), and treatment program admission that will enable cross study comparison and the potential aggregation of data. The second approach requires a systematic investigation of the influences on treatment admissions, particularly the substance abuse patterns and the ecology of treatment services. With the accumulation of data over the past decades such investigation should be feasible. Finally, we need strong theoretical models and heuristic hypotheses to guide future analyses and interpretations involving treatment data. The increased use of treatment data in a sound framework should advance not only our scientific knowledge about drug use epidemiology, but also help guide policy and practice to better address the needs of the millions suffering from drug abuse and dependence.

REFERENCES

Brodsky, M.D. (1985). History of heroin prevalence estimation techniques. In:Rouse, B.A., Kozel, N.J., and Richards, L.G. (Eds.), *Self-Report Methods of Estimating Drug Use: Meeting Current Challenges to Validity*, NIDA Research Monograph 57, NIDA, Rockville, MD., pp. 94–103.

Craddock, S.G., Rounds-Bryant, J.L., Flynn, P.M., and Hubbard, R.L. (1997). Characteristics and pretreatment behaviors of clients entering drug abuse treatment: 1969 to 1993. *American Journal of Drug and Alcohol Abuse* 23(1), pp. 43–59.

Gardiner, K.L. and Shreckengost, R.C. (1985). Estimating heroin imports into the United States. In:Rouse, B.A., Kozel, N.J., and Richards, L.G. (Eds.), *Self-Report Methods of Estimating Drug Use: Meeting Current Challenges to Validity*, NIDA Research Monograph 57, NIDA, Rockville, MD., pp. 141–157.

Greenwood, J.A. (1971). *Estimating the Number of Narcotic Addicts*. US Department of Justice Document No. SCID-TR-3, GPO, Washington, DC.

Levin, G., Roberts, E.V., and Hirsch, G.B. (1975). *The Persistent Poppy*. Ballinger Publishing Co., Cambridge.

National Institute on Drug Abuse. (1980). *Data from the Client Oriented Data Acquisition Process (CODAP), Series E, No. 18, State Statistics 1979*, National Institute on Drug Abuse, Rockville, MD.

National Institute on Drug Abuse. (1994). *The Washington, DC, Metropolitan Area Drug Study. Current Treatment Client Characteristics In The Washington, DC, Metropolitan Area: 1991*. National Institute on Drug Abuse, Rockville, MD.

National Institute on Drug Abuse. (1998). *Assessing Drug Abuse Within and Across Communities: Community Epidemiology Surveillance Networks On Drug Abuse*. National Institute on Drug Abuse, Rockville, MD.

National Institute on Drug Abuse. (1997). *Epidemiologic Trends In Drug Abuse, Volumes I and II: Proceedings, Community Epidemiology Work Group*. National Institute on Drug Abuse, Rockville, MD.

National Institute on Drug Abuse. (1996). *Epidemiologic Trends in Drug Abuse, Volumes I and II: Proceedings, Community Epidemiology Work Group*. National Institute on Drug Abuse, Rockville, MD.

Substance Abuse and Mental Health Services Administration. (1995). *Treatment Episode Data Set*. SAMHSA, Rockville, MD.

Substance Abuse and Mental Health Services Administration. (2003). *The DASIS Report* (May 30, 2003). http://oas.samhsa.gov/2k3/multiYr/multiYr.htm.

Substance Abuse and Mental Health Services Administration. (2004). *The DASIS Report* (April 9, 2004). http://oas.samhsa.gov/2k4/dualTX/dualTX.htm.

Substance Abuse and Mental Health Services Administration. (2004). *State Estimates of Substance Use From The 2002 NSDUH*, Chap. 5 http://oas.samhsa.gov/2k2State/html/ch5.htm#5.4.

Treatment Episode Data Set, 2002. http://icpsr.umich.edu/SDA/SAMHDA/04022-001/CODEBOOK.

Woodward, J.A., Bonnett, D.G., and Brecht, M.L. (1985). Estimating the size of a heroin-abusing population using multiple-recapture census. In:Rouse, B.A., Kozel, N.J., and Richards, L.G. (Eds.), *Self-Report Methods of Estimating Drug Use: Meeting Current Challenges to Validity*, NIDA Research Monograph 57, NIDA, Rockville, MD., pp. 158–171.

Index